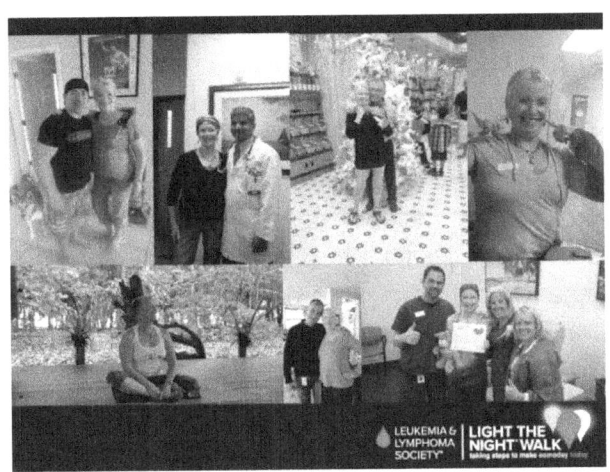

Chemo Saved My Life

Yoga Saves My LIVING

Healing the Mind & Body Through Injury and/or Chronic Disease

By

Faith Bevan

MS, PA-C, PYT, E-RYT 500, YACEP, C-IAYT

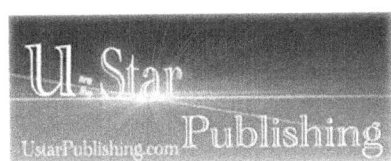

Dedication

Thank you to my medical providers, Dr. Uday Dandamudi who got me through diagnosis to remission with RCHOP, Dr. David Wenk who has been there to monitor me post chemo with repeat blood work and PET scans (and we need to talk about that one too) and the remission neuroses. No thank you is complete without honoring the wonderful people that work at the cancer center from those at the front desk who learn everyone's name to give them a welcoming smile, the schedulers who adapt and adjust to prescriber's directions and the patients efforts to have a life outside of testing and treatments and the infusion nurses who become such a vital part of our lives. They are the front line of our well-being, notifying the doctor when they feel something is amiss, holding your hand and being there as someone caring, listening to fears and tears, all the while following the prescribed protocol of infusing toxic chemicals into your body. Not a very positive environment for them to be in day in and day out, and I hope they are taught, practice and use skills for self-care.

My family and friends were there to support me, care for me and try to understand and accept the transitions in my physical and emotional being. My husband John worked at keeping us whole as a couple, making me laugh and taking me for Thai food on Saturdays (he really doesn't like Thai food so that was a big deal), my son Nick who still treated me as Mom, not sick Mom, and was there for me when I was afraid to be alone when my husband had to travel for business. And they put up with my germ fetish not wanting to touch menus, asking for water without ice or lemon, not touching door knobs or light switches and constantly using hand sanitizer. My friend and co-worker Kim who would bring me Tom Yum soup (my favorite), gluten free crackers, would go out on walks with me and drive me around to see patients. Always a smile and cheery face. And my neighbor Ingrid would check in during the day just to see how I was (I really think she was checking to make sure I hadn't dropped dead) and drop me off for chemo and my friend Carol (sister from another mother and father) would pick me up from chemo getting me a Starbucks Chai Latte (just 3 pumps, some extra hot water and soy milk) and take me home where waiting for me was organic vegetable soup, mashed potatoes and hummus – comforting food she had made for me. (I hadn't eaten mashed potatoes in years before this) She would sit with me until John came home from work and return the next day to sit with me until it was time for us to go back to the cancer center to get my shot (had to be no less than 24 hrs. since the infusion for insurance to pay), and then we stopped for another chai. (Carol confided in me later that her actions weren't totally altruistic but were selfish. She wasn't ready to lose me so she was going to see to it I did well. Love you Carol and Thank you my dear friend/sister) The good things in life are still good even when your health is challenged and maybe those good things are that much better. We shouldn't wait until something bad happens to appreciate those things.

And to those at Flow Yoga who stepped in to cover the classes, clean the bathrooms and floors, wash the towels, make sure everything ran smoothly, and all those who faithfully attended classes, followed my progress, dedicated classes to me, sent prayers, had prayer shawls made, gave special presents to soothe and comfort me. To know I had so many in my corner sending the best they had to my rescue. With love and gratitude, I can never thank you enough.

And on a somber note, to those who have become part of my life who have had not as good an outcome of their journey, treatment and life. Your source of joy in life, passions and strength have helped guide me, and have filled my heart with both love, respect and sadness. You will live forever in my thoughts and have provided me with wisdom and strength. Namaste

"Life is a journey that must be traveled no matter how bad the roads and accommodations."
Oliver Goldsmith

Ustar Publishing
7705 Grand Boulevard
Port Richey, Florida, 34668
www.ustarpublishing.com

Copyright @ 2018 by Faith Bevan

All rights reserved. No part of this book may be reproduced or utilized in any form or by any means, electronic or mechanical including photocopying, recording, or by any information storage and retrieval system, without permission in writing from the publisher.

Note to the reader: This book is intended as an informational guide. The remedies, approaches, and techniques described herein are meant to supplement, and not to be a substitute for, professional medical care and treatment. They should not be used to treat a serious ailment without prior consideration without a qualified care professional.

Library of Congress Cataloging-in-Publishing Data

ISBN : 1727174429

Printed and bound on demand through Amazon Create Space

Cover, text design and layout by Joseph Verola

To send correspondence to the author of this book, faithbevan@gmail.com

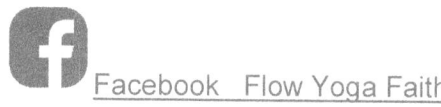 Facebook   Flow Yoga Faith

Index

Dedication 2

About Faith 6

To the Reader 7

My Journey of Healing Through Cancer to Living Life to The Fullest 8

Just Breathe 10

Our Nervous System 12

Let's Get Physical (My favorite Olivia Newton John song) 13

Section One 14

My Personal Journey 14

Post Treatment "The Scares" 22

Tools to Live This Life 24

The Journey Doesn't End at the Conclusion of Treatment 26

The Chemo Chronicles (This is My Personal Journal & Facebook Posts) ... 40

Section Two 72

My Tools of Healing Through Cancer to Living Life to The Fullest 72

Journaling 74

Nutrition 76

The Practice of Breath, Movement & Mindfulness 94

The Breath 94

The Mind 99

The Physical Body 103

Let's Start 104

This Isn't the End 115

About Faith

Faith Bevan lives in Port Richey, Florida with her husband John Cavaliere and cat Karma. She has one son, Nick Tumminello (Coach Nick), who is a well-known fitness writer and presenter. Owner of Flow Yoga in Port Richey, is a Physician Assistant, Professional Yoga Therapist-Medical Therapeutic Yoga, Yoga Alliance Registered Yoga Teacher and Continuing Education Provider, and a Certified International Association of Yoga Therapist.

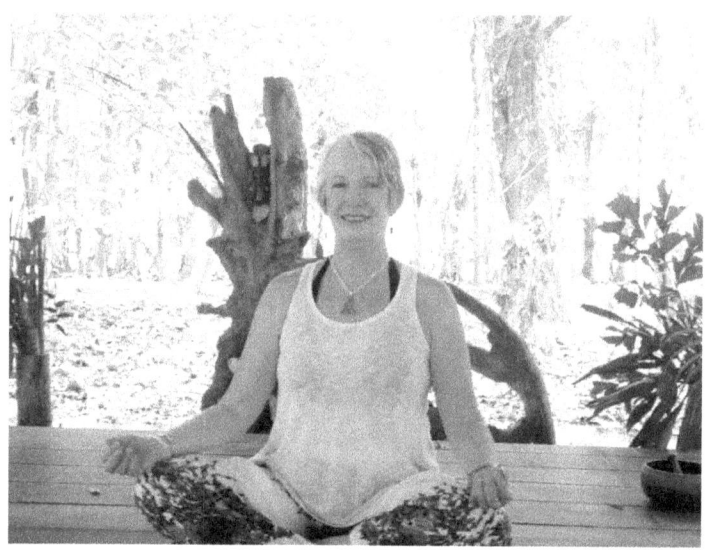

You have to accept whatever comes and the only important thing is that you meet it with courage and with the best that you have to give. **Eleanor Roosevelt**

To the Reader

We have no manual to life, much less a how to when told you have a life altering or life-threatening illness or injury. As a medical practitioner with over 20 years of experience I have seen my fair share of illness, injury and despair. And there is often little we can do except deal with the issues in a very clinical manner. I was unprepared to hear those fateful words it is a blood cancer. I'm here to provide you with some comfort and direction should you or a loved one must deal with cancer or another life changing/threatening illness.

I hope to share with you, about living and thriving while in the battle, caregivers and those seeking knowledge, the roller coaster ride from health to illness and returning back to health; the dips, the turns and screams, the terror and depression, and the tools that helped serve me every day. Don't wait till the bomb goes off, we need to have the tools, keep them polished and know how to use them precisely, because the time to learn how to use them is not in a time of desperation. That time is now, The Present.

This book is not a substitute for medical care and guidance. And share with your medical providers any information and tools for their approval before undertaking them. Written in Two Parts complimenting one another. For all who love, who breathe and feel; those who are well, are ill, have lost or loved; everyone is touched by illness or injury sometime; or maybe you are just on the roller coaster ride of life. There are no instructions, flow charts or manuals for life, so I chose to research, journal and document this ride, and now I am sharing it with you.

Part One: My Journey of Healing Through Cancer to Living Life to The Fullest

Chronicles the journey from health through illness and treatment, to remission. You will share in my fears, the tears, the smiles, the pitfalls and the growth; there is information, introspection and inspiration.

Part Two: My Tools of Health Through Cancer to Living Life to the Fullest

Shares information and tools, I found helpful to regain my life. An easy to follow guide on nutrition, meditation, breath work, yoga postures and movement. You don't have to be a yogi, just able to breathe and wanted to learn to improve today and tomorrow.

"Life is 10% what happens to you and 90% how you react to it." **Charles R. Swindoll**

My Journey of Healing Through Cancer to Living Life to The Fullest

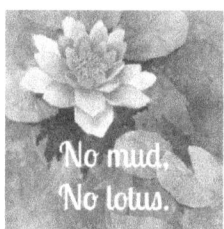

"You gain strength, courage, and confidence by every experience in which you really stop to look fear in the face. You are able to say to yourself, 'I lived through this horror. I can take the next thing that comes along." **Eleanor Roosevelt**

There is nothing that sends terror into every molecule of your being than to be told "you have cancer". We don't have to go far to be reminded of family and/or friends who we have lost to cancer or to hear of those with fame and fortune for one reason or another. It is no surprise that the initial response is "I'm gonna die" but of course we all are sometime. Like you have just been stamped with a best used by expiration date. But as someone in my support group stated so well, "But yes, we are all gonna die sometime, but We know what we are gonna die from."Ugh!

As a medical practitioner with over 20 years of experience in emergency medicine, internal medicine and mental health I have seen my fair share of illness, injury and despair. To keep myself healthy both mind and body I adopted a green diet about 40 years ago, avoided tobacco smoke even second hand and chemicals, limited alcohol to a wine socially and ate non-gmo and organically as much as possible. Kept a healthy weight, exercised, practiced yoga, relaxation techniques and meditation. Did everything right, had the tools to live a long happy, healthy and vital life. Not only did I blend the benefits of the ancient wisdom with that of technology (east meets west) but I taught and mentored others in kind. How blessed to be able to merge the 2, sometimes divergent philosophies, to see how there is a complement, an integration, as opposed to alternative.

But none of this prepared me for that fateful day in November 2014 when I heard those words it is a blood cancer. We will do more testing to find out which one and get you on chemotherapy. The idea of chemicals coursing through my veins was the LAST thing I wanted to do, and especially after I had proclaimed many times, "if I ever get cancer I WILL NOT do chemo". So, I was about to eat those words because I knew at how quickly my spleen enlarged and ruptured, this cancer was out to get me, its mission was kamikaze. If eating greens, alkaline diet, etc cured cancer, as some claim, I wouldn't have gotten it in the first place. I knew that the show was on, bring on the toxins, kill as much of me as possible so those suicide bombers get knocked out and hope that all that good living and those tools that I had will revive me and return me to wholeness. This is the ultimate betrayal, your own body, your cells, your DNA programmed into destruct mode - yikes.

So hard to accept this reality. Many people at this point ask "why me?" I always felt many cancers are caused by random mutations without the normal cancer-causing associations so why not me? But I had hoped those mutations wouldn't be happening unless there were other unknown pressures on the body causing them; why would my lovingly cared for body going into destruct mode.. So, I was searching for the why in a more cause and effect way. That medical, scientific, analytical mind just searching for an answer. And I have always felt there is power in knowledge, tell me something and I will question it, just not the one to just accept things as truth. Because in this situation you are powerless to the terrorist take over and with some understanding maybe I could snag it in its game.

My hematologist/oncologist was a super guy, smart, direct, kind, caring, great bedside manner; and I owe the guidance to my medical remission to him. I was blessed to get him and I am so grateful to him every day. But what about my emotions, my fears; my life isn't about statistics; luckily, I had a 50-60% chance of going into remission and I meditated on that, used affirmations with that, but I wrote my obituary just in case. Funny thing about obituaries, are they saying what the person would have wanted people to know, would they have like what it said. So, I decided I wanted my obit to reflect the legacy I hoped to leave. I was never offered mental health counseling, only given books about chemotherapy, diet (not what I felt were the best and healthiest food choices-stuff I wouldn't eat when healthy), side effects, etc.; and the photos in the book were always people smiling. That isn't happening, it's BS, you have to really dig deep to smile, and laughter forget it. Like those muscles, the part of your brain that says happy is in a coma. Just as in dying and grief there are stages, I now know there are stages in the cancer journey (same holds true for any serious injury and life-threatening illness) and I am still learning about them as time goes on, as the journey doesn't end with remission, it just takes on a different essence and flavor.

I hope to share with you, about living and thriving while in the battle, caregivers and those seeking knowledge, the roller coaster ride from health into illness and treatment, then returning to health; the dips, the turns and screams, the terror and depression, and the tools that helped serve me every day and to this day. Don't wait until the bomb goes off, we need to have the tools, keep them polished and know how to use them precisely, because the time to learn how to use them is not in a time of desperation. It is Now, The Present !

Just Breathe

The first thing we do when we are born is take that breath, and the old joke "wanna live a long life – well just keep breathing". So. our first and most important tool is our breath. Sounds crazy, of course we are breathing, it is automatic. But our respiratory system is the only system in our body that is both autonomic and voluntary. Think about the last time you got a scare; your breath became shallow and rapid. This sets off a cascade causing more stress and anxiety, releasing a cascade of hormones that target every organ system and cell of the body. The brain waves become erratic and the cycle keeps going, the sympathetic nervous system (fight or flight) goes into full swing and the last thing you can do is think clearly. We can intervene through our breath and redirect this process to help us keep our calm and sanity. We will learn about these techniques later on.

Let's look at what can get this process going. *Number One is fear.* Fear of what is going to happen to me, of losing control, fear of losing your job or your life's savings, fear of putting a hard ship on our family, fear of losing our independence and being reliant on others, fear of pain, fear of the effects of the treatment like losing our hair (even in the face of illness we still care about how we look), feeling ill, fear of being alone, and fear of dying, and I could go on, we can just keep adding fears to the list. And fear is a calm word, perhaps it really should be terror. Because from that day forward your life is forever changed, you are changed, how people look at you is changed, think about you and treat you changes. Your identify changes both within yourself and to others, and sometimes we feel we don't recognize ourselves. And the fear doesn't resolve when you hear the words you are in remission; Because the fear then becomes a persistent whisper, a twinge, a sensation, whatever it is-It is There. I call it the suicide bomber stalker. Attack is imminent, when least expected, just like it popped up out of nowhere, nothing to keep it from returning.

The next is denial. In denial we can become complacent, depressed, avoid making decisions that can be crucial to the outcome. And frequently leading to the worst of all, doubt and distrust. We doubt that our efforts of treatment will be worth it. How can we trust ourselves when our bodies have defied and betrayed us? How do we trust the doctors, the medical system as a whole, and big pharma, and what about the conspiracy theories withholding "real cures"? It is funny how we want to believe the infomercial type of articles and sales pitches about "real cures", but yet we distrust and doubt research and verifiable and reproducible results. Now I'm not saying that the medical community is giving promises, in fact all they can give are statistics, studies. etc. but at least there is something to back up what they say. And we all want a miracle, to defy the odds, we put on a happy face for others but the self doubt resonates deep. If there truly were a secret, a "real cure", is it reasonable to think we would never find out about it and it become the "cure". We are in an age of technology and fast communication, what do we not hear about almost as soon as it happens???? I doubt anything could be really kept secret.

"Proof is boring. Proof is tiresome. Proof is an irrelevance. People would far rather be handed an easy lie than search for a difficult truth, especially if it suits their own purposes."
Joe Abercrombie

We experience a huge sense of *sadness and anger*. And you have a right to have those feelings, whether you are facing it yourself or you are facing it affecting someone you love and/or care for. Nothing makes people feel angrier than feeling out of control and helpless; their life spiraling out of control, picking up speed with no stop in sight, having to put your trust and life in the hands of others creates a huge stress response and this one presents even more problems as it can make us unwilling to being accepting and compassionate to ourselves and the condition. And anger at others especially when they say well meaning but inconsiderate things such as think positive, or you look good (and you are thinking "pretty good for a dying person") or tell you about someone they know who just died from cancer (like I really want and need to hear that). And then, of course, they tell you all about the miracle cure or how deadly chemo is they read about on the internet. What do you say, thank you for making my day! Let's just say anger over the stupidity of it all.

And let's not overlook *Desperation*. When we grasp at anything and everything, regardless of how crazy it may sound. It is that looking for the magic, the miracle, even if the medical treatment is showing good result the endless quest. Even if a medical remission is achieved, the desperate search never ends. The doubt that the remission is real, the fear of relapse never leaves. The desperate desire to be free, cured and no longer belong to that club that bears the insignia of that disease. The endless state of being on guard for that suicide bomber stalker to rearm, strategize and launch another attack. This is anxiety, this is stress, the thoughts just come in even though we are commanding them to go away, we feel the muscles in our body tense, our breath becomes restricted and that cascade takes us away to a place that is painful both mentally and physically. Many people will take anti-anxiety medications, and believe me, they have their utility, and sometimes just getting knocked out is what you need; but when it wears off you are still there in that same place. And the anti-depressants can help us too, but the reason for the depression is still there. The worries, the stress is still following us everywhere we go. So, we need tools that we can access anytime, anywhere, without harmful side effects. And that is our breath. Long slow sweet savory breaths, nothing switches our nervous faster than the breath. And add a little sigh to it, just feel the muscles melt. Ahhh!

"Our bodies are our gardens – our wills are our gardeners." **William Shakespeare**

Our Nervous System

There are 2 components of nervous system that we will discuss here, the sympathetic (fight or flight) and the parasympathetic (rest and digest). We have the 2 operating all the time to keep our body and organ systems balanced but when we are in a constant state of stress, and even during out fight during treatment and healing, the sympathetic can go into overdrive. Vagal tone is considered the key to finding balance and restoring us back to calm. Studies are showing how we lose this tone with the stress. PTSD (post traumatic stress disorder) is not uncommon with people who sustain a serious injury or illness, it isn't just from trauma like what is found with the military. The body responds to stimuli/stress and goes immediately into that stress response and loses the ability to return to calm. This can be triggered by a word, a smell, a sight, a sound or just the body not recognizing that the threat has gone or isn't real. The scary thing is this is a primitive brain function whose function is to keep us safe. It remembers what is dangerous to alert us. But sometimes it won't stop alerting us or it doesn't shut itself off sensing danger everywhere, even when danger may not really exist

Think about the last time you were in the car and you thought another car was going to hit you, that near miss. Your heart raced, you gasped and then held your breath, and then you felt shaky. You felt short of breath and maybe even sick to your stomach, maybe even began to shake, you felt a sense of doom and discomfort, but suddenly the body realized the threat had subsided and before you even recognized the change you were back on your way as if nothing had almost happened. When you lose that vagal tone it just doesn't go away and your senses are heightened, to be hyperalert and hypervigilant, expecting the attack and ready to fight or flee. But, when it is an illness, an internal threat, you can't run away. The threat is you, there is nowhere to go. This is something that no one will tell you about, so it can be quite frightening and very unsettling. And what makes it even more scary is it may happen later when you think you should be feeling better, a delayed reaction that can make it even more difficult to handle. And you think it is just you, but I have heard this from almost everyone I've talked to.

"There's so much behind my smile you just don't know. Everyone sees who I appear to be but only a few know the real me. You only see what I choose to show." **Unknown**

Let's Get Physical (My favorite Olivia Newton John song)

Our self-image, self-esteem and identity really takes a hit when we sustain an injury whether it is a short term or long-term process, and when we are diagnosed with a life changing or even threatening illness. Ask a runner about how they handled an ankle sprain or a yoga teacher with a sore shoulder, unable to do the activities they love and schedule their life around. This sounds trivial but it can have a significant impact on someone. It wrecks your identify, and we take it as though we are being punished, your life many times is wrapped around those activities and now EVERYTHING is put on hold. And we aren't even talking about a devastating injury with that either, but now consider something that is life altering and/or potentially life ending. Perhaps surgery changing the body, never to return to its previous state, or the deterioration of the body from the disease itself like loss of strength, or the effects of medications like weight gain, and we all know the effects of chemotherapy with hair loss and neuropathy. How do we learn to accept what is and find a way to love ourselves even when we despise what has happened or is happening to us? We want to be like we were because that is where we are comfortable but we will never be there again. To still honor ourselves, to care for ourselves lovingly, to forge a new identify and sometimes having to find new meaning and new purpose in life.

These are not things the docs will tell you about; and quite honestly, are disconnected to. There are books that talk about caring for your skin, make up and wigs but that is what is going on on the surface only. They can give you the side effects of this and that, offer you antidepressants, urge you on by telling you how well the therapy is working. But in the end, only you can make the shift. Having the awareness comes first, ceasing to look at ourselves as parts and pieces, and connecting to our wholeness, taking a holistic approach to healing, being our true selves. It is the work we need to do to not just be survivors but "livers" living, loving, laughing and embrace our beautiful gift of the present. Whether we have many presents ahead or a few. Make each moment count, live it as it is the last for you or maybe for someone else important to you. We only get one shot at that moment.

"The present is our gift, there are no exchanges, refunds or credits." **Island Style-Key West, FL**

"There are moments when troubles enter our lives and we can do nothing to avoid them. But they are there for a reason. Only when we have overcome them will we understand why they were there." Paulo Coelho, The Fifth Mountain

Section One

My Personal Journey

As a healthcare professional I had not taken any special interest in cancer care, as far as I was concerned if I find something I just refer to the specialist. And once the patient came under the care of the cancer center I didn't see them much. So, except for the clinical aspects of my diagnosis and illness I was truly clueless. And I'll admit to you that I wrote my obituary as I had a preconceived belief about cancer treatment and the outcome. (*yes, I had said in the past, I'll never do chemo*) Luckily, I was open and willing to eat my words and go for it, chemo and all. And afterwards, I certainly didn't have any trouble saying, I was uninformed. (**Belief:** the state of mind in which a person thinks something to be the case, with or without there being empirical evidence to prove that something is the case with factual certainty. In other words, belief is when someone thinks something is reality, true, when they have no absolute verified foundation for their certainty of the truth or realness of something. Another way of defining belief is, it is a mental representation of an attitude positively orientated towards the likelihood of something being true.)

From Never Sick - To You Have Cancer

I noticed fullness in my abdomen I was in diagnostic mode. Running through a differential of diagnoses seeing what other symptoms I had and how was it impacting my activities, appetite, work, sleep, and yoga. When I felt I needed to alter my movements while teaching a yoga class on that fateful Saturday I knew I was in for a big deal. When I got the CT and blood test results I once again ran thru the possibilities but then blurted out, "It's a hematologic malignancy". Game on, which one, will it be treatable, how much suffering will I experience and will I die quickly or a long drawn out miserable process. The medical mind vs. the be in the present, focus, one step at a time, and breathe. There was no sense of panic, no tears, just a feeling of numbness. An odd thing happened the evening before I went to the hospital. (My cat Karma for the first time ever brought a rat into the house, ate it under the bed and then left the remnants there.)

So, in the hospital I was equipped with my relaxation tools, eye pillow and calming music. As I waited between specialists, blood draws, visitors, I propped the pillows behind my back to form a supported yoga pose, put on my eye pillow and found my breath. I transported myself from the sounds of the hospital, the cold unforgiving environment to a peaceful still inner space. I knew that I needed to be open to what was ahead no matter how painful the reality was. The Yogi/Physician - give me the facts, no sugar coating, the clinical in me needs the facts, the yogi needs to go within, one is outside research and the other is introspection - inner evaluation. Going thru the resources, the catalog of thoughts, sensations, and events. My past-what went wrong, I was strong, vital, healthy, vegetarian for 36 years, ate organic as available, loved, laughed, took care of myself, no stresses other than what just being alive gives you. Always feeling grateful and trying to find the best in every situation. OMG, I maintained a sense of calm and inner control taking the immediate not looking beyond. But I was sure my spleen was going to rupture and at that time I was more concerned about that immediate consequence, internal hemorrhage, shock and surgery. This wasn't the medical person but the person who has a lot of awareness. I could feel the changes however imperceptible they were to my outward persona, lack of pain, physical exam and vital signs, I knew and told everyone "it's going to blow". Intuition, awareness, fear, whatever it was, I knew. So often during my medical career I would just know, was it the hairs on the back of my neck standing up, that gut sensation, can't say, it is just there, the knowing. And long ago I learned to trust it.

It ruptured and the journey to emergency surgery was surreal. The phlebotomist who came to draw my blood for the type and cross was someone I hadn't seen forever. We were both happy to see one another but not in these circumstances. When I was wheeled into pre-op it was like an angel appeared before me. It was Patricia, a nurse I've known for years. Her words were I'm going to take good care of you. I love you. And when I awoke from the surgery 2 more angels appeared, one was Pat one of my personal training clients, who worked post op and the other was Kim my ARNP business partner and friend. The universe called in the recruits and they answered the call, they came to the rescue. I was surrounded by the light of love and support. It wasn't until weeks later I realized the hematologist/oncologist that was on call that day would save me not just from the cancer but from myself. But all the while a sense of calm, no sense of doom. The medical person awoke from surgery asking how much Morphine, Versed, Propofol, how many units of blood? How are my vitals, Kim was laughing as I recited how much of each drug I received before I went out, my brain still on-on-on. It was a fight for my life. One step at a time, be in the present, and now I have become a medical consumer, not the deliverer of medical care. I struggled to not give up control. Medical Consumerism Sucks!!! I always said there is more healing on the yoga mat than in the medical visit. Game on, walk the walk, not just talk the talk. Control, what do we really control, we think we have it all covered, but suddenly it comes down to this moment. The more out of control we are the more we try to control.

The first post-surgical day in the ICU was a drug haze. I was aware but disconnected and that is scary. Monitors, IV's, catheters, I wanted to breathe, to move, again be in "control". Not much to do but try to make sense of it. They check your vitals, ask you questions but with the drugs, it is all a garble. My experienced mind knew what was going on but all the brain functioning was so dulled. On Day 2 post op I was eager to reconnect to me, I asked them to stop the drugs and that is when the healing began. They were suspicious about my not being on the strong IV opioid pain killers but for me that disoriented/disconnected feeling was going to be a hindrance. Most people are calmer and still on the drugs, but for me they just made me want to fight. I had a 10-inch incision running from the base of my sternum to my pelvis, wow And I was so swollen up, I felt 8 months pregnant. #1 on my list, yoga, to start the opening and clearing process; pillows, blankets, everything I needed to restore and to renew. Work on the breath, get those lungs to open, keep the chest open, the mind open. Deep breathing is paramount, as they give you an incentive spirometer for you to work on the breath, but yogic breath work, same thing you just don't need that plastic gizmo. Breath, life, love, gratitude, survived this first hurdle. Must be open to what comes next. Stay in control, watch, wait, find focus, stay calm. No tears, just the job at hand. Get out of the hospital alive. Day 3 gotta get out of the bed, need my healing pose- downward facing dog. The neck can't turn as there is a central line, gotta guard the large abdominal incision, but something magical about the downward facing dog, a perfect balance between strength, stability, focus, calm, and letting go-nirvana. In the pose the body finds the place where everything lines up and lets go. Hands on the bed, slowly walk the feet back, extend, soften, breathe, feel the energy and life moving into the body. AHHHHH I am alive and living again is before me. I can do, I will do, I will heal, Yoga, move it, breathe it, feel it. And tears began to pool in my eyes, because at that moment I knew I was going to live. The magical Zen moment was interrupted by a visit from my oncologist, I thought he was going to "shit". "What are you doing?" My answer, "I am healing". There were some other words of disagreement, and disapproval, but that didn't stop me. Day 4 I got moved out of the ICU and into Telemetry, I continued my breath work, they monitored my incentive spirometry-made goals, I exclaimed "yoga". I was moving in and out of the bed better and better, turning down oral pain medications and not because it wasn't painful, as it was, but I had tools, couldn't twist because of the incision but could do hip openers. Hands on the chair, squat-breathe flow. Does the bowels good! That was another eye opener for the nurses as I am in goddess pose (a wide leg squat) with a hospital gown, central and peripheral line and huge abdominal bandage. Did I mention the smile - bliss on my face! The medical person could give all physiology of the trauma, healing, rehab etc, but it is the yogi that began to heal from within. Listening to my body not to the fears, being willing to explore the "now" and not having expectations. Enjoy the journey, the new path that life has taken. A time of learning. Accept change.

"We must let go of the life we have planned, so as to accept the one that is waiting for us."
Joseph Campbell

One week after going into the emergency room I was discharged home. The first thing I wanted to do was roll out my yoga mat but I knew I was going to have a tough time getting down on the floor and then back up. So, my bed had to suffice. Pulling my knees to my chest never felt so good as my body could sink into the pose with a complete release. (Apanasana/Release Wind Pose-about letting go what doesn't serve us) I began some low gentle bridge poses; however small they were they would transport me from pain to pleasure. And began the smallest of twists, using the pillows and contour of the bed to support my body and prevent too much twisting in my belly. I would retreat back into the bed frequently during the day to find my yoga. And it wasn't long before the beckoning mat and I reconnected. My mat stay unrolled in place for 6 months, blankets, bolsters, blocks, ready for me at any moment as I knew this would be my magic carpet ride. I was getting Home Health visits 3 times a week, they would find me in a yoga pose and I must say I've never seen so many jaws drop. I had a different nurse for the 4 visits with them, all 4 had to double check how many days post op I was. They were amazed. I always had a smile, stated that ALL body functions were just fine, only took something for pain to sleep, as I had no pain as long as I could retreat to the mat when I needed to. I was moving with a sense of freedom and I was less than 2 weeks post op but was doing a downward facing dog with my hands elevated on a block. As long as I could suspend myself there all things were possible. I followed up with the surgeon 2 weeks to the day after surgery with a big smile on my face, I moved freely and even he had to double check how long it had been since the surgery. The healing of my incision was great, I moved without pain and counseled him that Yoga was the path. He felt that there was nothing I needed him for, I had gone farther than expectations so he discharged me and said call him if I needed him. I asked him when I could go back to teaching yoga classes and he said if I felt up to it go ahead. I thanked him for saving my life and my next adventure was yet to unfold. Since I was feeling so good I was sure that what happened was a fluke, it couldn't be a cancer after all. Surely, I was healthy, as I was healing at a rapid pace and quickly regaining my strength. DENIAL!

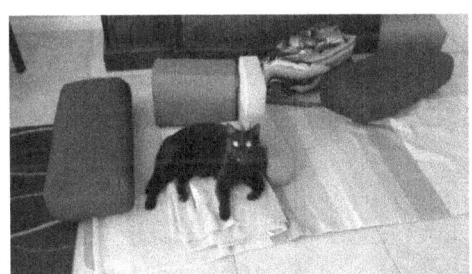 My cat Karma kept my mat safe and warm for me.

I had a follow up appointment with the oncologist that same week. It was my first appointment at the cancer center. I don't have words to tell you what a sickening feeling it was signing in there and going through the process. There was an air of misery and desperation; I felt sick in the pit of my stomach as it hit me-Not a club I want to be a member of. He, too, was surprised and thrilled at my recovery. I reminded him of his concerns with my yoga in the ICU with a little smirk, he just nodded. What could he say!!! Little did he know that wouldn't be the last of my "You need to listen to me". At this point I felt like a victor, I am well, it is gone, I am going to be fine, certainly I can't heal like this and have a suicidal demon plotting and rallying inside of me. And, yes, the preliminary pathology concurs, it was a marginal zone splenic lymphoma (lymphoma only in the spleen), the spleen is gone and we will wait and see, usually no treatment is necessary. But to be complete we should do a PET scan, even though all the CT scans I had in the hospital were negative for any other evidence of the lymphoma, no lymph nodes seen in the chest abdomen or pelvis, just the HUGE spleen. But the PET scan looks for metabolic activity, the hallmark of cancer, this will be what we will use to monitor the disease. And, of course, was I excited about MORE radiation, up until then I even avoided dental xrays. Between the time of that appointment and the PET scan a few days later I developed some very strange sensations. The best I can describe it is like having a truck scooting around my body, stopping to make a delivery. I swore I could feel the lymph nodes pop, but no discomfort, no pain, just something odd was happening and it wasn't good. I would press, push, and search for something, anything and then suddenly there it was, a palpable lymph node in my neck. The following week I saw the oncologist, he told me the he was sure all was well, my blood work was better, I had healed so well, looked good, felt good. I told him of these odd sensations and he shrugged his shoulders, I then said it is throughout my body and he went thru his check list, fevers, night sweats, weight loss ……. The answer was no. Then I told him how I knew, as if the odd sensations and node wasn't enough, but I had attended a gong immersion a few days before. I felt a dullness in my body where usually the gong would resonant throughout and when I was reciting to myself affirmations of health it appeared that the gong vibration was bouncing off and away rather than being absorbed by my body. I am sure he was thinking, "I have a real crazy one here". And then he finally looked at the PET scan. To hear your oncologist, say "oh shit", you know you are screwed. Now this is when He needed yoga, as the pathology said one thing, the PET scan said another, this is really bad. The reality really hit here, I am going to die, I must prepare, must get in control. Breathe, Cry, Breathe. Get everything in order, this is how the story ends. Be present, be focused, can't control this but continue to breathe as long as I can. Write the obituary, make sure all passwords and accounts are organized. John needs to know where everything is, can't depend on me anymore. Make sure my end desires are known and will be carried out. My best friend keeps saying don't think like this, stay positive. Not things to say to someone told they have cancer, don't know what it is as the pathology is obviously wrong, and has moved throughout the entire body in 3 weeks. Stage 4, the worst in blood cancer. Not good. Must do more yoga for living, as long as I can, breathe, focus and be present for this part of the journey. It isn't about healing now, it is about just breathing and living, staying calm til acceptance. Should I call Hospice now?

I tell the oncologist if we don't get this figured out fast I'll be dead in a few weeks. He says "don't say that" with a sense that he now realizes I am completely in touch with my body, I have his complete attention. Because things didn't correlate I needed a new biopsy of a very large lymph node behind the liver, I am referred to the hospital but they won't do it, referred to someone who will do it via EGD (a tube down the throat into the GI tract) but they can't see me for 2 weeks. I'll be dead by then. More yoga, listen to calming music, breathe, stay calm, acceptance. Gotta love Facebook, I put this out there and a friend of mine (a former yoga student), an Interventional Radiologist, says call me I'll do it. He knew things weren't good for me and he threw his hat in the ring. As opposed to the hospital, he did it in the office so I wasn't sedated, just local. Very uncomfortable but gotta do it. He went thru my liver, got the node and success. Another angel came to me, their nurse Mary. She and I bonded as she stayed with me for hours as I had to lay on my right side to keep from bleeding internally. My blood pressure was up then down then down even more but eventually it stabilized and I went home. Carol and John were there at my side. Carol was rubbing me with lavender essential oil, and John went to Starbucks to bring us our sustenance

A week later, Christmas Eve we had the answer, now we knew what we were fighting, a very aggressive deadly lymphoma, not good but makes sense. I say Ok let's get the drugs going right now and they say can't do that. Sounds crazy to me and they ask me why not wait til after the holidays. Are you kidding me? I'm gonna be dead by then, or at least a lost cause. Now I want it now, best they can do is day after Christmas. But there is another hurdle, can't start chemotherapy without an echocardiogram as one of the drugs can be toxic to the heart. It's Christmas Eve no offices are open, can't get an appointment will be dead by the time we get it. So, I phoned a friend, a former yoga student is the wife of a local cardiologist. I called her and guess what her husband told his echo tech to wait for me. Echo is done, and heart is good; on Dec 26 I begin chemo. Thank you, Dr. Rao Musunuru,

After I had the echo I went to my hair dresser; it was just a mere month ago, I had my regular appointment, color, trim, style. I cherished my long reddish-brown hair. Wore it down, up, straight, styled – my signature. Hadn't had short hair since elementary school. Thank you, Shawn and Angel, for easing me into hair loss. My bestie Carol came with me as I got a cute short stylish do. When it started coming out, the last thing I wanted were long strands laying on the pillow, this way I was giving up my hair, I wasn't losing it.

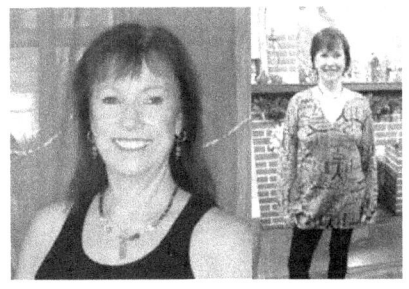

"Don't just learn, experience. Don't just read, absorb. Don't just change, transform. Don't just relate, advocate. Don't just promise, prove. Don't just criticize, encourage. Don't just think, ponder. Don't just take, give. Don't just see, feel. Don't just dream, do. Don't just hear, listen. Don't just talk, act. Don't just tell, show. Don't just exist, live." **Roy T. Bennett, The Light in the Heart**

Treatment Time

As a yogi, someone who cherishes wellbeing, does all the right things to stay healthy, chemo is completely at odds. Poisoning my body; it goes against everything I've done, know and believe. But then gotta remember there is a suicidal demon dancing inside. How and why did it get there? I prepared for the chemo by reading everything I could about how each one worked and, of course, the side effects, and the side effects, and more side effects, and some side effects don't show up to years later. But what choice did I have - acceptance! Acceptance of imminent death or acceptance to go out kicking and screaming with poisons coursing thru my body. Acceptance, be present, be strong, breathe. Denial was gone, reality isn't pretty. "My last supper" was with my husband and best friend at a Thai restaurant eating the spiciest soup I could. I knew it would be my last for a long time and maybe the last ever, as once I began chemo everything would be different. I prepared a poster to accompany me to chemo, I would become a Warrior, *Warrior I - a powerful way to build concentration, balance, and focus. It creates strength in all areas of life — physical, mental, emotional, and spiritual. Practicing this pose regularly will help you to face the challenges of daily life with equanimity and poise. Beyond the physical posture, Warrior I creates deep concentration. Focusing on your foundation and building the pose from the ground up reduces distractions and hones your energy. Your mind becomes focused, calm, and clear.* - Exactly what I needed. This, a prayer shawl made for me to keep me warm and protected, a stuffed cat given to cuddle became my constant companions, my intention in my practice in my breathe in my life. In the morning prior to chemo I would sit quietly and meditate, try to calm my anxious mind listening to some healing chants sung by Snatam Kaur, do some Sun Salutations (a series of poses that invigorate the body and prepare you for the day. It is about preparation, use the tools, and don't forget to Breathe. As I would sit in the infusion chair my poster sat by my side and I would sink into the awareness of the poisoning process; Inviting it in as a life-giving elixir. Looking at the poster I would connect to the Warrior in pose and words, reconnecting to my inner strength. "I am a Warrior, strong, focused, capable. I am victorious in this battle, I am a warrior." At the end of chemo, I felt like a beaten warrior but the next day was a new battle. That was a time for restoring, my body, beaten, weak, and aching. I would allow my body to find its stillness on the mat with the support of the blankets, bolsters and blocks. The breath returns, no time like right now, that is all there is. Gratitude for making it thru to this moment. Need air, sun light, life around me, so walk, walk, walk. Breathe in life, acknowledge the cancer cells decreasing in number and tell them their days are numbered, regaining health and wellness. Moving meditation, a walk of life, living, breathing and being. Recent research with mice showed that exercise helped distribute the chemo, get it everywhere, the more the better, yay. Visualize the cancer cells going into a wood chipper and being ground up into inert particles and then cast away. As the days progressed my poses grew, the Warrior took a stand, dizziness took over, hard to walk without wanting to hold on to someone but move slowly, linger, savor, breathe.

Search for strength, patience, focus, honor the body even though it is defying me. Believe Believe Believe, don't give in. Sleep is allusive, strength fades, bald isn't beautiful and when the lashes and brows went, it really set in. Eye liner, blush, earrings and scarves, make a statement, I am alive. I warned everyone, when I don't put on the makeup or jewelry you know it is time. I find patience in holding yoga poses, if I can hold I can stay "powerful". Don't give in, is it your mind telling you you're weak or your body. Breathe, focus, be present, the Warrior. But it was a time I felt vulnerable, how does a yogi have to hold on tight walking down stairs or be afraid to take a walk alone. Anyone please walk with me, stay with me, I am in Fear.

"It is better to light a candle than curse the darkness." Eleanor Roosevelt

Post Treatment "The Scares"

Elation when you get the results that you are in remission. This isn't a get out of jail card, just a reprieve of unknown duration. I then truly become a "cancer survivor" (the term is widely used for anyone diagnosed with cancer and alive) as while I was immersed in the battle I considered myself a "cancer fighter" but a whole new set of issues come in. This is when I became anxious and depression would creep in. Crazy, you now have a you are clear, and now you develop issues with anxiety, panic and anger; makes no sense. But while you are receiving treatment you have a team of people seeing you, rooting for you and supporting you. You live from test to test, treatment to treatment, measure to measure. You are so intertwined with the external manifestations that you aren't within yourself. And when you are done you are on your own. How do others do it??? I have my breathe, my focus, awareness, my mat always there for me, my practice and I am suffering. It is with you always, every ache, sensation, thought. It's like a stalker always lurking and threatening to show up when you least expect it. I've understood depression, anxiety and PTSD at a clinical level but now it's at a personal level. The heart starts to race for no apparent reason, a sensation of overwhelming fear, without a focus, it is just there. I can't sleep, I would peel my skin and body away to get away from this horrible feeling. Instantly angered, ready to battle, doesn't matter what it is; because everything else is trivial-I just went thru chemo, could die any moment, I hurt, I'm weak, cry.... Breathe, eye pillow, listen to Yoga Nidra. I am now teaching again and my calm is on the mat always. I try to share the wisdom of this journey, as my personal practice has deepened and how important that connection is. What I have learned and the small successes are the biggest. I am rebuilding strength, balance and endurance, but the body rarely is without discomfort somewhere. This part of the journey has its own essence and direction. Become whole again, just live, make plans, and become not just a cancer survivor but a liver. Even if there is only 15 mins to spend on the mat spend it. Time spent nurturing the self is the best time spent. I arise each morning with whatever little sleep I got glad to see the day, grateful for all the opportunities I have had in the past and the opportunities I have before me. To truly be in the present, be true to myself, and acknowledge what is. Acceptance no matter how unpleasant or painful and breathe. In this journey I have really learned the meaning of the real yoga begins off the mat. The mat is where we learn and practice but our life is where we live our Yoga.

It is important for us to have the tools for our life before we need them. We need to know how to use them, to keep them polished and the tool box accessible for us. We practice today for what may be tomorrow. I may still have survived the process without the yoga but I don't know if I would have really lived during the process and now. I kept my mind, body and spirit vital, was able to reach up both physically and emotionally when I needed and to know when to ease in and out of both poses and circumstances. Yoga, Life, Have Mat Will Live.

But even as time goes on little changes, oddities about the body can persist. Who would know, the hair is grown into a stylish do, the eyelashes are coming back donning lots of mascara, fully engaged in life, work, physical activities. But the "weirds", little electric shock like sensations that come out of the blue mostly affecting the legs, moving up, down and all around, they come out of nowhere. Disordered sleep, a few hours then awakened hourly, and any noise resulting in a startle response preventing sleep all together. Get that jumping feeling going. When the nervous system gets going it just doesn't want to turn off, the anxiety has me pacing, walking in circles, doing my breath work but the body feels like it needs a strong jolt to get it to stop. And then there is muscle and tendon pain, totally strong, lots of endurance during the activity but afterward, my body thinks it is running a marathon every day. I figured I was hurting without doing really exertive activities so I tried running again, started off amazing, slowly building the distance, getting my stride and in fact the muscle pain lessened. Ha Ha, it was then my knees and ankles yelled out "Arthur Lives Here" and he is pissed off. (Arthur of the Itis family) Well, my few weeks of running joy and feeling of LIFE, I ended up with weeks in pain walking, moving. Tried it again, and again, and again; each time same result Yes, I did hear that chemo progresses arthritis, and did I find out it's true big time.   They say chemo ages you by 10 years, yes, I feel it.

This is living the "new normal". And some tell me that in ways they see things about me that are better. I do not want to waste time or energy on the trivial, and I definitely don't want to be "uncomfortable". In the past I embraced challenges, physical and mental, but today I feel I survived the biggest challenge of all, the fight for my life. But I also don't want to miss a sunrise or sunset, the sight and sound of birds, the purr of my cat, Karma, the kiss and touch of my husband, John, and the chance to talk to my son, Nick, and enjoy hearing about his endeavors and successes.   A definite deeper appreciation of life, nothing to be taken for granted. That doesn't mean I don't like adventure, but I'll just plan it in temperatures and places I'm excited about.

"People grow through experience if they meet life honestly and courageously. This is how character is built." **Eleanor Roosevelt**

Tools to Live This Life

1. Acceptance   This situation, why fight the obvious, when we accept What Is we can rally our energy where it needs to be. As much as we would prefer things to be different, they aren't, so go with the flow, paddling against the current a hard and disappointing road to follow. This doesn't mean giving in, it means giving ourselves permission To Be and go from there.

2. Get Help   Enlist assistance of friends, family, support groups, counseling, and ask your medical team. This is a time when flying solo isn't the best route to take. This is about making your life about living every moment.

3. Find Joy   Even in the most miserable situation we should try to find a sliver of joy. Whether it is meeting someone, learning something new, or seeing something that brings a smile to your face. Look into the sky, see the sunrise, listen to the birds, smell a flower, whatever it is, you are here, enjoy the ride no matter how bumpy it is.

4. Find Meaning   Why are we here, what is the purpose of living, Your Legacy?????   Perhaps you can help someone, just with a "I've been there", make a friend or mentor someone. Write a book. ☺ Love, Laugh, LIVE

Relationships

When illness or tragedy strikes each individual, the patient, family, friends, caregivers, is hit with their own set of issues, trials, fears, desires, losses, strengths and weaknesses. For some, bonds are strengthened, some are challenged, some are frayed like a rope giving way from wear but continue to function and some disintegrate under the strain. But not just the strain of the illness or treatment, time constraints and financial burden, but of the loss of what was, the change in identify, abilities, outlook on life. Nothing can change you more than meeting your mortality, fighting for your life with every breath and speck of energy you have, and then continuing the fight every day to preserve what you have, to mourn and accept what has been lost and to try to find peace with the new normal.

Caregivers can become exhausted caring for someone, often neglecting their own needs, and usually not by choice but out of need. Lack of sleep, social contacts and isolation only worsen the depression that frequently accompanies illness of someone important in your life. Children can have difficulty in the role change, and when a parent is ill may find themselves being less than accepting of care. It isn't an easy path and being ill isn't a time to let ego get in the way.

This is really when you find out who your real friends are. If you can no longer go out and socialize, maybe have dietary restrictions that make going out to eat a challenge or just not be up to lots of activity that very much needed friendly interaction can wane. And when we are ill, we frequently have all our time wrapped around going for tests, getting treatments, seeing doctors etc. so we may not have so much to offer in conversation. So those that are just for the good times may fade into oblivion and become part of the past. And then some will step up to the plate and be there for you, loving you, supporting you and being the shoulder to cry on, the one to share your fears with. And they come back day after day, because they are there for you not just for the good times. They are your past, your present and will be the future.

In the case of a significant other or spouse it can strengthen and bond people together or create a crack that deepens into a fracture. When one faces illness and especially a life threatening one, the other half may be forced to look at their own life, purpose and mortality. That can be an earth shattering and home wrecking experience requiring a lot of soul searching and introspection. Sometimes, the changes in the daily life, activities, adventures and intimacy can cause a fracture that culminates into a relationship split. The one with the illness struggles to survive, to find acceptance and peace with the new normal, but the partner may resent the loss of what was and what has been changed and lost in their life. And then there are those who reconnect to their partner, rekindling their bond and love creating a renewed joy in the partnership and lives. And there are those who ride the tides of change like a surfer, on for the joy, fall down, get back up and do it again, enjoying and savoring each part of the adventure.

I have been fortunate to have a wonderful friend, Carol, I call her my sister, who nurtured me throughout the journey and beyond. We are luckily now back to girlfriends getting together and having fun.

When my mother died of cancer, I was there for her in the last few weeks of her life, she was under in-home hospice care. Until then she lived with her husband on the other coast of Florida from me in the winter and back in Baltimore the rest of the time. I would visit as much as possible but never served as a caregiver and being physically removed I never saw the day to day until the final days. And even then, we had the in-home care so I could be the daughter and not the caregiver. But the other day I saw a friend who had recently lost her mother to cancer, my friend is a nurse going to school for NP and her husband is a radiologist. With them both being in medicine, to hear them describe being primary caregivers to her mother for 8 months and how this has reframed their view of practicing medicine, patient interactions and their own emotional state. These are 2 people who are financially and emotionally stable, can get whatever help they need and they are suffering. Trying to regain their life, reconnect to their relationship and shed the stresses of caregiver. All I could think as we talked, the toll is even bigger than anyone can imagine and there is no structure of care out there to help the patient and their survivors. So, I offered to her, as I am trying to do, is let this experience show you the way to reach out to others, there is no learning more than experience, and using that empathy that comes from the deepest part of our being, to lead the way to help others.

The Journey Doesn't End at the Conclusion of Treatment

As one of the worst days of your life is hearing you have cancer, a joyous day is you are in remission. But with that comes the words just go live your life and we will see you back in 3 months. So of course, the question is asked, "what can I do to keep it from returning?? – the answer is NOTHING". And each and every day it is a wonder, a worry, a question of am I fatigued, what is that pain, is that a lump, OMG I have a headache (must be brain mets). Time goes on, we get back into life, work, recreation, can eat out again without the concerns of being immune compromised, travel, hopefully many of the chemo side effects start to fade and eventually resolve. And for some they treat you like you are a hero, how they admire your strength and perseverance, but in reality, you put on a happy face because no one wants a moper, a complainer, a downer. But the fear is so real.

For myself I found community in a cancer support group. We had all ages and types of cancers as well as stages. We all understand that there is something special about the journey and only someone living it has the understanding. When family members, care givers accompany them to the group you can hear the contradictions, frustrations and lack of understanding. One man's wife kept saying he wasn't trying and all he could do was tear up because of the pain he was in both physically and mentally knowing he was letting her down, but he couldn't make her understand. And I'm sure that he kept having to be reminded of what he had lost in life and the prognosis for his future was not something he relished.

I've heard some say that it was the best thing that ever happened to them, yikes, that is pretty scary but it does reset your life, your views, your vision, your relationship to self and others. You always hear the phrase "don't sweat the small stuff" and wow, that is so true. You realize just how insignificant our day to day trials and tribulations are, how we get all worked up over little stuff, meaningless stuff, stuff not really worthy of our time, attention and certainly not our stress and anxiety. It is a time to step back, reassess, gain a new appreciation for the present moment. To set goals for the future but not to put things off til tomorrow because you realize tomorrow may not be the day you planned and wished for. To stop and smell the roses. I remember many many years ago, when someone asked me if I ever stopped to smell the roses, I gave a nasty egotistical retort that I owned the rose garden, all was in my control as it was there at my disposal. How I have learned so to the contrary. That the rose garden is all around us. We move at such a fast-frenetic pace we pass it by, overlooking the beauty and joy that surrounds us, that fills our life. We close ourselves off from our senses, of smell, touch, sight, and go thru life with blinders on overlooking anything on the periphery. So, to feel that this is the best thing that ever happened is a bit intense, perverse and scary but it is definitely transformational.

Do we embrace the change, not just accepting who we have become with all our flaws, our strengths and changes, or do we welcome it and truly go with the flow? Learning to explore the new me, to learn anew shedding the old skin, the old ideas and hang ups. I so often hear people ask "when will I get back to like how I was" – the answer is NEVER. We don't go back, we go forward. We are forever changed in mind, body and spirit. And if we ask why me, we get stuck in that question, because it is not why me, it is why not me. It is about setting our course to live our best life possible, but just like when you set your GPS it always has the "rerouting" option when taking another turn or path. We need to continue to grow in intellect, compassion and empathy on this journey. L'chaim (to life)

The first thing I did at my heme/onc appointment after my last treatment was ask if I could travel. Spending 6 months in what felt like a cage, going to treatments, having blood draws, seeing the doctor, counting off the days until I could expect to feel a little better, the chemo affects begin to wear off, avoiding public places and crowds because of germs, touching things etc. I needed to get away, to just feel normal, to have a life that didn't revolve around Big L. (as I unaffectionately call it) and medical appointments. There was a YogaFit Mind Body Fitness Conference in Minnesota coming up and it had been my goal to attend. I wanted to see my friends who had supported me through calls, emails, song and videos and to expand my world through learning things unrelated to cancer subject matter. Stagnation in mind and body isn't living, it is just existing, and during that time of treatment you have a sole focus of getting it on, over with and then on with living. Smelling the roses, laughing, loving, LIVING. Receiving the go ahead I booked the conference, hotel and air. I notified friends across the country in hopes they would be attending and those who put on and teach at the event I was coming home. Because that is what it felt like, a homecoming; coming home to myself, Faith. The craziest part was I was so psyched, I totally had forgotten how to travel, about checking in 24 hrs before (and I was flying Southwest so that is important), I was the last to board but that was OK. When I went up the escalator to the gates at Tampa International Airport it felt like it was the very first time I was going to fly, I was overwhelmed with a wave of excitement and emotion. And as I rode the escalator I was crying my eyes out, not sadness, not fear but "I am here, I am alive, I am doing this. If you had said to me 7 months before I would feel like this I would have told you you were crazy, I flew all the time, no big deal, like brushing my teeth, but this was so different. Last to board, I took out antiseptic wipes, cleaning the seat belt, arm rest, tray table, then the essential oils under my nose to decontaminate the air I was breathing, and an extra dab on my hands to cup over my face if I hear any coughing or sneezing, just in case. I had become neurotic about the worry of germs and getting sick, even the thought of catching a cold was still terrorizing.

I settled in, did my usual counting of seats to the emergency exits, sizing up the people around me who could be an obstacle to getting out in a crisis situation and who may require help, and then feeling grateful for being there. As the plane began to take off I tuned in, as usual, to the sound of the plane, feeling of speed, watching the ground move away and feel the gentle lift off from the ground, communicating in my head to the plane "fly baby fly". At that, I began to sob uncontrollably because it was me spreading my wings again, flying, not just in a plane but in life. I was taking off to a new adventure, to places unknown in my own body, mind and soul, a new me, a new direction. I truly had been given a chance to start new again, a new path, and I was prepared to embrace everything that was there for me to see, feel, taste and experience. The conference felt like a coming home party, a reconnection to who I was, I was there hanging with friends, making new ones, and I was honored by Beth Shaw, the founder of YogaFit, it was a truly amazing, inspirational and experiential weekend. Thank you to my YogaFit family.

As many people who have a life changing/threatening situation do is make a bucket list, all the things you want to do before you die. Fortunately for me there isn't a lot on that list but one thing is I wanted to do was see whales in the wild. So, I chose to go on an Alaskan cruise with my husband, son and his then girlfriend, and my best friend Carol and her husband. Cruising is my favorite form of travel and definitely the best if you are traveling with others, lots to do, always know where to meet up, and everyone can do what they want for themselves. We went on a whale watching boat in Juneau and we saw humpbacks and orcas. OMG, again the tears, I was so choked up, same thing happened when we were at the Hubbard Glacier, tears, lump in my throat. My son looked at me perplexed, he had never seen me emotional like that, we had been to MANY places, been on many cruises but never crying. Had to explain to him the fact that 8 months prior I didn't think I would be alive much less experiencing this. He heard it and nodding oh I get it, but no he really didn't. Because for him he saw his mother who was dancing, hiking and working out, not dragging around but ready for the next adventure even though sleep was still eluding me.

My live life train wasn't stopping but all the while I had a hard time making commitments, I knew what I wanted to do, where I wanted to go and when, but this little issue of is it coming back kept creeping in. I had always been a person who said, I want to do that and I did. Now it was if I pay the money what will happen if .... Yikes. Went to MD Anderson in Houston for Yoga for Health – Integrative Oncology. Part of me hated the fact that I understood way too much of what they were teaching, and another part of me was very proud to be knowledgeable about the subject matter and sitting there to explain it from a personal perspective. I was there not as a patient but as someone who knew this stuff really works. All steps putting life together, renting a car, getting myself to and from the airport in a strange place, may not seem like a big deal but it was, a little chemo brain disrupting sleep, some small memory issues and body aches, but doing it and getting on with it.

A few months before I headed to Houston I saw an ad in the Tampa Bay Times for the Suncoast Chapter of the Leukemia & Lymphoma Society Light the Night Walk scheduled the following month. I put it aside at first thinking, "if I'm alive I want to do that". But things started looking pretty good, had a clear scan at my 6 month follow up, I was back to work, getting stronger physically but still struggling with insomnia. But getting over the frustration of not being able to sleep, getting into the acceptance mode and going with it. (definitely understand why sleep deprivation is a form of torture)   That fundraising even turned out to be one year from the great spleen adventure, I raised a little over $1,000 for the cause, and when I went to registration and they asked if I was walking in support of someone or in memory of someone I said "in support of me". I was then sent to the survivors' tent and when they handed me the shirt saying survivor on the back, I got choked up, started to cry – AGAIN. I cried more in the year post diagnosis than I did during it all. I looked at that word "survivor" and there are no words to describe how I felt, both uplifting and depressing.   It was a funny thing not long after that event I started to communicate with them and then they asked me to be the 2016 Honored Hero Survivor. I told them I was no one's hero, but I would be honored. I thank them for making my living affordable as they paid a lot of money on my behalf during treatment.

December 14 is my wedding anniversary and my wonderful husband John said let's go on a cruise out of Tampa and have lunch at our favorite Mexican restaurant in Cozumel, Casa Denis. Not one to ever turn away a cruise, but there was a bit of irony in it. When I got diagnosed one year before I told my husband that I wanted him to take my ashes on the Royal Caribbean ship out of Tampa to Cozumel, have lunch at Casa Denis, be sure to dance with my ashes at the disco and make sure he got to hit all the spots I always enjoyed. And then to sprinkle me in Cozumel, all around the ship, and in the water while at sea.   For both of us this was definitely a much better deal. ☺ We had a great time and except for my now having short grey hair it was, laughing, loving and LIVING.

We spent New Year's as we had all the previous years with my son and his girlfriend in Lauderdale, we missed 2014 there but he and his then girlfriend came to spend New Years with us.   That New Years I was sure it would be my last so when I got to be part of the celebration I was yahoo yahoo, I really did make it. Funny how those milestones are so significant but always tinged in a sense of doubt and trepidation. It is like having some say something positive and then say but if this or that. To say this all messes with your head is saying it lightly. I feel so fortunate, though, to have a wonderful son who likes for us to spend New Years together, I always tried to spend it with my own Mother, so it is the one holiday that means a lot to me. And now it is sooooo significant, an achievement, like receiving an Oscar for Best Performance in Living.

I treated myself to a big celebration trip, again I had wanted to do it, but hesitated to commit because of the lack of confidence that all would be well. Luck was on my side, there was a room in one of the houses, as opposed to a tent, at the Professional Yoga Therapy Institute's first annual retreat at the Costa Rican resort Boca Sombrero. A week living on the ocean listening to the waves serenade me at night, getting comfortable being in the open air, as there is no in-door or air-conditioned space, the toilet and shower facilities are downstairs and outside. High end roughing it, as I was never into camping even as a kid. I like Hyatt's, and the creatures, oh my.

But it was pure heaven, I went on the river hike, never was much for that, never was a rock skipper especially in moving water, but wow. Saw poison dart frogs, toucans, lots of monkeys, and at the house the iguanas during the day and all the bats, huge beetles and roach like critters. And, yes, I slept in a mosquito net, and they sweep every day the wood pellets from the termites.

But anniversaries were on the horizon, one-year anniversary of having the PE, of hearing the words no sign of lymphoma the PET is clear, of the last chemo and of stepping out of what feels like being in protective custody of the Cancer Center into the scary world of what now. Knowing a blood draw and PET were scheduled, anxiety began to grow, my intelligent mind kept saying you got this, you are OK, working every day, exercising, dancing, living a normal life, except, of course for that damned insomnia; but the emotional anxious mind is scanning for trouble, anywhere in any form. It isn't realistic, it is being neurotic, a fear that just comes over you like a character in a horror movie that keeps jumping out of unexpected places. And when I talk to others, others who are 5 years out and more, say the same thing. So, I guess it just goes with the territory. One gal in our support group said it like this, everyone is going to die of something sometime, but we know what we are likely going to die from or with. And this is it, we all know that every time we go out on the road we or a loved one could be involved in a fatal accident. So, none of us know what the future brings, but with this it is like having an expiration date that has been extended to date to be determined.

At one-year anniversary. PET and blood work 6 month follow up, Blood work not perfect but nothing alarming for the doc, I'm alarmed. Funny, I used to evaluate every number, every statistic, but now I don't, I know that an elevated LDH will freak me to the max, so now unless it is a change to where I stand treatment wise la la la la la. At one point I asked the doc if my elevated LDH's weren't going to change anything, not get me on the road for stem cell transplant or put me back into some form of treatment, why get it. So, he agreed that he wasn't going to order it. For me the elevated LDH made me feel like a sniper had me locked in as a target with a laser scope. So not ordering it again made me feel better, because what he was saying it is nonspecific and he wasn't worried about it was likely true. My LDH was high at presentation and all during treatment except for the very last when it went down and started increasing again after treatment. I was convinced that it signaled impending doom, but so far that hasn't been the case.

Just as that first trip to the yoga conference heralded my freedom, I decided to embark on an adventure that always appealed to me. I decided to go on a transatlantic cruise, 13 nights aboard ship, only 4 ports visited once it crossed the Atlantic. And the best part was I planned on going alone. My intention was to get a lot of writing done, spend a lot of time in reflection and healing; and as much as I love my husband, he and I have such a good time together, I wanted this experience alone. It was almost like I needed to re-establish myself as an independent, capable, resourceful and healthy person. Of course, there is nothing challenging about the adventure physically, all the comforts and even more, but I was alone, would I be lonely, get neurotic and depressed with all the alone time or would I be able to be outgoing and meet people, engage in interesting conversation that didn't center around the "journey". The first night aboard ship made me fear it was going to be a long lonely 13 night. It seemed to be ALL couples, was I the only solo traveler? I decided to not go to the dining room, my long-time travel agent had me at My Time Dining, I never liked MTD and had asked her to have me at early seating so I never checked. Yikes, all I could think of was going into the dining room and sitting ALONE, so I opted for the Windjammer doing a quick grab, eat and go. I then went to the lounge grabbed a glass of Prosecco and asked myself "what were you thinking?". I had cruised many many times before, I began cruising with my son when he was 17 and when my husband and I got together he then joined in. So, I've never been on one alone, was always a family affair, a fitness or yoga cruise, or one with family and friends. And about the Prosecco, before I had chemo I enjoyed red wine. But once the chemo was done the mouth dryness lingered and that it was an issue, it started to subside but it wasn't gone. Red wine just didn't taste good, felt burny and unpleasant, but the cool sweet bubbly of Prosecco became a special treat. And because most people drink bubbly to celebrate or on special occasions, I figured it was quite appropriate, as my living was something to celebrate – Everyday. Turned out I met a number of others who were cruising solo, and did it on a regular basis, so what was I thinking this was a biggie. For some a form of emancipation and others just like it that way. I enjoyed it so much I booked to do the same the following year. Knowing that you can cancel without penalty up to 3 months before the cruise I felt like I was safe booking, just in case. I was able to get a reduced deposit amount and $200 ship board credit, so was too good to not do it. And if I made it to sail the following year, yes it would be time for celebration and more Prosecco.

At the other end of the TA cruise I met up with my son at Heathrow who flew in from Florida and we then flew onto Milan to connect with my husband who had been riding his bike throughout Italy. We took trains from town to town, walking constantly with luggage from train to hotel and back, walking all over Milan, Florence and Venice, climbing the stairs of the Coliseum and the Forum in Rome and stairs in and out of metros. Every day I had to check in and remind myself of the activity I was participating in, being free of fatigue and weakness. Wow, it finally clicked Faith was back and I was shedding that identity of the year before. Not quite as dramatic as a snake slithering out of their skin all at once, but this was slow, little bit at a time, til finally, voila, telling myself I was healthy I could finally say it with full conviction – I'm believing.

I got a cold, not really a bad cold, pretty mild in fact, but left me with a runny and swollen eye for a few weeks, in fact that eye thing started while I was in Italy. I've had that before, years ago so I didn't associate it with anything other than the normal upper respiratory stuff. The eye cleared and a few weeks later I felt some odd sensations about my scalp and head. I started to focus in on it, Is that a headache? Is it sinus? Is it in one place? Is it a mass in the brain? And as luck would have it I attended at this same time a Pain Medicine conference in Orlando and one of the lectures was on headache. So of course, there was a case study of a woman who had been treated for breast cancer and went to a headache specialist for headaches. With her history they were concerned, scanned her head and she had mets in the brain. From then on, the neurosis returned big time. I was constantly mentally scanning and analyzing my head sensation. Did it resolve with an Aleve, a Tylenol? Would a brain cancer headache be relieved that way? Oh shit. I couldn't think of anything else, I didn't mention it in group, I certainly didn't mention it to my husband until one day he asked me what was wrong, I guess my trying to act "fine" gig wasn't working. I got a MRI of my head/brain and all was clear. The headaches magically disappeared. All my energy, focus and worry about the headache actually made the headache persist. Definitely a mind body thing.

At this point we are well on our way into the fundraising for the LLS Light the Night in November. My mission is to educate the doctors, the nurses, the financial counselors about LLS and to make sure the patients have access to their information and contact. LLS even made up business cards for me so I share them eagerly, but it really is interesting to reflect how I have taken this crappy situation and turned it into a mission. Guess it is that make lemonade out of lemons thing – well maybe that is why they gave me that part to play. I have had a few patients referred to me by some doctors to talk to and help, but we really become partners in the process. Gives me a sense of purpose to now be on the other end of it, now finally feeling like I've accomplished something staying healthy, living life, and loving every moment of it. Someone told me that it never goes away having that little voice, that fear, but you just don't think about it as much; it doesn't intrude on your quiet time, your fun times, your loving times as it does at first. The words of affirmation recited numerous times a day are there without the feeling that something is sneering behind the curtain laughing.

I now go to scan and blood work time again feeling cocky, I am healthy, I am well, nothing to be found here, and then the lean in. You know when your medical practitioner leans closer, lowers their voice and says we see something …………… and oh shit. Can't be, I am healthy, I am well, no weight loss (please!!!!!), no fatigue, no lumps bumps etc, I am active, EVERYTHING is fine, just got some pretty nasty seasonal allergy stuff going on-yes that is what it is seasonal allergies. You know the stuff healthy regular people get. Well, turns out there is up take at the left nasopharynx not seen in previous scans. And then the words "I'm not worried about it, we'll just rescan you in 3 months to see if it changes/resolves". And my answer to that is "no we won't-I'm going to the ENT and let them directly scope it and take a biopsy". I've had more than enough nuclear material and radiation into my body, so doing an extra one is not acceptable. And I had just had a MRI of my head, brain, sinuses a few months before and that was clear. He looked at me so perplexed, and then said, "well, if that is what you want to do". And I said hell yes, so to the ENT I went, he did a direct visualization, I started sneezing like crazy, he didn't see anything he felt needed to be biopsied and stated you have allergies. He then said I'll see you in 3 months and we will take a look again. Now that made sense, no nuclear crap put into my veins, no bombardment with radiation, an annoying but not painful office procedure you walk out from, no fuss no muss. It's not just about PET scans are limiting to no carbohydrates for 24 hours before and complete fasting for 12 hours before and no coffee either. And then laying there motionless in that long tube for 20-30 minutes, nothing about it is what I want to do any more than I have to. And why do they think just waiting and rechecking is acceptable. I have told the doc, you don't get it, you don't have a friggin clue; I get the stare back and then the response, you are right. OMG!!!

Life before cancer was really so simple, get up and do my thing, whether that was work, seeing patients, teaching yoga, personal training, or personal life of family, friends, socializing, housework, shopping, traveling. Never a thought about illness, obstacles or negative outcomes. Life has hurdles so I always felt they were there to challenge me, to never be complacent, to always tap into the adventurous and inquisitive side. And how to learn to truly go with the flow, why fight what you can't change but put your energy where it can be productive. Caring for people with illness was my job, I knew the medical side of things and except for being with my Mom for the last few weeks of her life I was never a caregiver. I felt with my Mom's illness my medical knowledge kept me together as I could look at things clinically with an understanding that would override my deep emotional pain. And while she was ill it worked, when she died I kept it together until I walked into the funeral home and I locked myself in the bathroom crying uncontrollably and inconsolably. My father died before I was in medicine, I was a young mother but I had an innate sense about what was going on, and he went quick. We had been to our usual Thursday lunch date and Friday night his heart said I am done. Except for my uncle dying around the same time as my Father, the only people I lost were grandparents, seemed right, they were older, that is how life goes. So. I was blessed with living and playing in the rose garden of life.

But now, the people that die are my peers (my cancer peers, that is), and each one is a wake-up call, a knock out of a hard-deep sleep, just when I am getting life back on track. The longer I live being free of that miserable stalker Big L I am back in that rose garden, life is awesome. Health is good, fit and active, riding my bike, teaching and training, traveling, no real obstacles to doing what I want to do. And then I hear it, someone is not responding to treatment, someone has passed away, and I am not sure if I am being woken up out of a dream or being put back into a nightmare. Throughout this cancer journey I never once asked why me, but in this survivor/liver journey, when I hear of someone not as fortunate I am finding myself asking "what is it about me and not them". I never understood survivor's remorse, and I wouldn't go so far as saying I have that, but I certainly have some uncomfortable feelings, questioning and not sure how to act, why me. People will say it's my attitude, my diet, my healthy lifestyle……. Blah blah blah, and I say, "I just got lucky". But I am not going to change all the good stuff I do for myself because it isn't just that the chemo worked, but I haven't suffered with a lot of the negative residual effects. Energy is good, sleeping has improved, my husband is thrilled that I am now riding my bike (as he thinks all problems can be solved by bike riding). And as I've been saying it is about living. I

CANNOT assure that I won't have to go to battle again, but I CAN say Life is Great, and it has all been worth it.

I do question when the fear will subside getting blood work and seeing the heme/onc in checkups. Can I not look at the results, dissect them, compare them to previous, evaluate every little nuance, I need to just hear the words, everything looks good and I go from there. My issue with the sinus had cleared up when I had it rescoped, as I knew it would; I am not fatigued, no night sweats, no lumps/masses, and certainly no weight loss-all the cardinal signs of a blood cancer. I ride my bike for 40 miles, I challenge myself to sprint 20-21 mph and I'm still questioning, evaluating myself, always asking "am I OK?". You NEVER go back to the way you were, it changes you, and I'm not talking about the hernia that has popped out from my spleen surgery. It is like having the alien from the movie Alien 😊. And it isn't about the gray hair, and, yes, I look at myself and say how old I look, but when I'm working out, teaching, riding, challenging myself physically and mentally, it is that voice that has a permanent implant and its name is fear. But I'd like to say some things have changed for the better as well.

A gal who comes to the Yoga Studio from time to time, but not regularly, was telling me that she was hoping to retire in 2 years when she turns 66 and then she would be able to come to yoga regularly. We started to talk and I couldn't help but go into my story of going from health and vitality to gonna die in a few days, no warning, no drawn-out symptoms, boom. And I told her I might as well been hit by a truck because that is how quick and hard my life as I knew it came to a halt. By putting off taking care of yourself, helping to limit your stress, just do things that give you joy, happiness and a generally good feeling, isn't the best decision. Why do we put ourselves last on the list, we tend to put everyone and everything else first, and if we are on the list at all we are at the end, if anything, if any time is left? It brings us back to the speech when flying, if the cabin loses pressure the oxygen masks will come down. If flying with a child or someone needing help, put the mask on yourself FIRST. This really is so simple if we don't save ourselves first how can we ever take care of others, or that huge list of things we expect to accomplish. So why I am now unapologetic to say no or I'm going to do this that or the other.

There is an old saying, and I have no idea who said it but "The only constant is change". And, wow, how right this is. We are changed every day from who we were yesterday. And most of the time we go through life never really thinking much about it other than when we see the signs of aging, weight gain or notice a change in performance in some area. Our identify may remain pretty constant most of our lives, perhaps we have always been athletic, or bookish, outgoing or even shy. When we experience a life changing or threatening injury or illness that identity takes a huge hit. A friend of mine, a dancer, figure skater and fellow yoga teacher, tore her Achilles tendon, we discussed not just the injury, the healing and the activities she is still able to do, not able to do and the alteration of her life. This hit her, her spin, her lift, she is still the same capable, beautiful, amazing person but it impacted her sense of self. What she expected of herself, who she was, so even for those who are introspective, reflective and honoring can have an effect on their life.

So, when I received my diagnosis I was no longer Faith the PA, the yoga teacher, the wife, the mother, the friend, the animal lover, but I took on the identify of a cancer patient. I can remember so clearly my first appointment with the oncologist out of the hospital sitting in the waiting room and stating to my husband that this was not a club I wanted to be a member of, and I was not happy. As the time went on, getting treatment, my identify became the bald woman wearing makeup, jewelry and coordination of clothes and head covering to try and look alive, living and not just sinking into the bald funk. I would put on my work out clothes and knit cap trying to be an identify that I wasn't dying but I was still living, just having the bad part of me killed off. And then when it was announced I was in remission I became a survivor, another identify, and then people called me a hero. I have never figured out how someone who has merely been lucky enough to have the stuff work and live through it is a hero. So, identify changes and now I am longer in remission, a liver, every day is a gift.

So recently I had a few things that challenged my "self" and I really couldn't understand my reactions and feelings. But after some introspection and meditation I think I may have some insight. I have osteoporosis so I have a fear of falling and breaking a hip. Not an unreasonable fear considering thin bones and my age. I'm back riding my bike and to give myself a greater sense of control and security I went from using regular peddles without clips so I can remove both feet without any hang ups getting my feet trapped. To enjoying a new lower profile bike decreasing my chances of not being able to catch myself in a mishap. When we were in Costa Rica recently I didn't try surfing, never really something I wanted to do as I thought falling off the board might not be fun (I do paddleboard, it is the being thrown down from the waves), and I opted not to do tree climbing, again not something that excites me. I did go hiking in the rainforest and guess what, I fell, my foot slid as I was walking across rocks in the river, never been my strong suit. As I was falling I thought "oh crap" and tried to lean forward so my knee would get it first and hip secondary. Success, I scraped and bruised up my knee but nothing was broken. The thing that was injured was my pride. I'd like to blame it on my sandals or any other variable but the reality is I just suck in those situations. I didn't like walking across logs, thin bridges, walking on ledges etc.as a kid.

Living in Florida it is warm almost ALL the time and when it is cool that's about it. No ice, no snow, no treachery, you just put on a sweat shirt, wear socks with your sandals and you are good to go. Since moving to Florida in 2002 I've gone up North only twice; the first time there was a dusting of snow and it was such a novelty, the second time was for my Mother's funeral in February 2006 and I haven't gone up since. When I see a conference or some event that looks interesting I opt not to attend if it is during the winter in the North. So, what was I thinking when I registered for a Yoga Therapy Symposium in Montreal in March. Well, I thought March can be warm, never been to Montreal, oh how bad (cold) can it be!!!! The week of the conference it snowed, a big storm covered the entire East Coast, shut down cities, airports, etc. I started to freak, OMG, I am supposed to fly up there. Am I flying, how much snow, the temperature said to expect 6 degrees Fahrenheit, you have got to be kidding me. All I could think about all week before I was to depart was the temperature, the snow. I am not one to pack ahead of time, but this took thought, wool socks (I have one pair), sweaters (I have a few), the one pair of corduroy pants, I do have a coat I purchased when I went to London years ago, and of course I have knit caps, wore them all the time to cover my bald head. When I moved to Florida I kept a token of cold weather clothes, just in case, but why have lots of it when it just takes up space and never gets worn. This completely took over my life, I became a nut about it, you would have thought I was being sent out alone in Greenland to fend for myself. I vowed that I would get a cab from the airport to the hotel and cab from hotel to airport and just stay warm and safe in doors the rest of the time.

It was cold but I saw the energy, the bustling activity on the streets, the people were walking fast thru slush, snow and ice. They were bundled up, had the perfect boots and were living their life without missing a beat. So here is what I discovered as I walked in the 20 degrees F, my eyes running from the chill, my finger tips cold in the gloves, my legs chilled from the knees down and my feet chilled in my thin bought them in Florida boots. But my, trunk was warm snug in my 3 layers, scarf and coat and it came to me. I was challenged about my comfort, my fears and my identity. There is nothing more uncomfortable than sitting in a chemo chair and having horrific poisons being pushed into your veins, the taste, the smell, the look, the ugh feeling, and then knowing you must keep going back for more. You find whatever you can within yourself to say "this is good for me-it is my life elixir". So, I just didn't want to be uncomfortable, I like hot showers, I rarely go in our swimming pool because I feel it is too cold, I much prefer the hot tub. So being cold, no thank you, actually hell no. And not just the planning to keep from feeling cold but what about cancelled flights, getting stuck in airports etc. discomforting just with the anticipation. And we know that only 10% of what we worry about ever is reality, crazy stuff. And then fear, walking in snow, slush, ice, what if I fall, I could break a hip. And not just that that would be bad enough, but then I would have a long recuperation, another identity change and then what would I lose and how would I come back. Fear can have positive effects, if there is real danger fear can keep us safe, alive. But this unrealistic fear, its crazy stuff. The biggest part of the fear, tho, was having to transform myself again, I've just gotten my life back into full swing. I forced myself to go out in it, nothing worse than missing out, and for me it was invigorating, like I faced a demon. Now I will tell you I have no intention of moving out of Florida but I MUST force myself into step out of my comfort zone. I am now very indulgent to myself traveling and doing everything I want, within reason, the thought of leaving my warm fuzzy has been out of the question. But I need to work on finding the comfort, the sweet spot in the discomfort, and make friends with it. It's not that I've become a spoiled brat that only wants things her way, it is I am allowing myself to be controlled by the fear, the unknown, the potential of having to create another new identity. And perhaps my fear is elevated because it is blood work time again and that is unsettling knowing that I can go into the appointment feeling fine and being told there is something concerning on the blood work and the sense of game over. Oh well, must take responsibility for myself, I am better than that. I hope.

And then there is being on a plane with people coughing, and I am quite uncomfortable about that. I use my EO sanitizer, Doterra On Guard, but I am feeling like there are all these hateful germs all around me, snearing and attacking. For the next 72 hrs, the incubation of the common cold, I will be vigilant of any signs of infection, not that there is anything I can do about it. I will take a bunch of Vitamin C and D as soon as I get home. And in 72 hours I hope to be celebrating I escaped. That neurotic thing again.

Back home, I enjoy the warm temperatures, I am the last to ever complain about Florida heat. And If you saw me riding my bike you would never think anything was ever amiss. I ride strong, have good endurance and can get a decent cadence/spin. But when I stop my entire body seizes up, and not just the legs, but the arms, shoulders, back, everything begins to feel stiff and rigid. I can hardy lift the bike to put it on the trunk rack and getting into the car is challenging. And then getting out, it is absolutely crazy, nothing wants to work. I take magnesium, quercetin, vitamin d and other natural anti-inflammatories and things to help muscle energy, but nothing seems to matter. Like the residual sleep disturbance, melatonin, valerian root, passion flower, chamomile, lavender, lemon, ocean sounds……… you name it – it's crazy. My John doesn't understand, it is a problem, he offers his ideas for it, but it is what the chemo did to me, something I can't explain. So, I remind myself "You are strong, You are capable, You are well, You got this".

Follow up appointments are a constant fact of life now. Goes like this: Doc asks/I answer: fatigue-NO (can't sleep well/always feel sleepy but different than fatigue, in fact strong and energy good); night sweats-when warm only but not the cancer soakers; lumps/masses etc-NO; weight loss-PLEASE. I fidget in the chair, let's get on with this perfunctory crap and to it. I say to him, having cancer really messes you up in so many ways. He then said to me "You Had Cancer". I recall the horrendous feelings I had going to the cancer center for first time and saying "not a club I want to belong to". And although I will always be affected by it, I am now an inactive member of the club. Living life and no looking back.

Wow, how does one react when you hear a partner in NHL is losing the battle, been through a number of different protocols and Big L is still attacking full force and gaining ground. As I herald my health, my renewal, I know that someone is preparing for the final chapter. How can that be that for me, one try, first pass and bingo. Is it the diet, the yoga, the affirmations, the acceptance, who knows, and we will never know. I feel guilty and I now pose that question "why me?" I never questioned why me when I was sick, but why me now. I am no better than anyone else, I don't have anything more valuable to offer the world, I'm just Faith. There are those smarter, richer, younger, and maybe more in a position to get any treatment out there to them just because of who they are, without good results. I am conflicted in being a beacon of hope, a testament to taking care of yourself and treating yourself with love and compassion and someone who made it just by being luckier than the next person. I am not trying to apologize for this but I am very humbled by it. Yikes, another one of the lessons from this journey. And when I speak to others who share with me their story of it from long ago, I know that sharing in the success of their healing is what it is about. I continue with my hemp oil and seeds, moringa, turmeric and eating a plant-based diet local and organic as I can. I am now taking a "medical food", methylated folate and vitamins that lower the homocysteine (a marker of inflammation), with my other healing vitamins/foods; donating time and money for the LLS, traveling, meeting people, laughing, loving and LIVING.

It doesn't mean the battle Is over, it has just changed. This is what I have to look forward to if Big L the suicide bomber stalker doesn't get me. Patients with diffuse large B cell lymphoma (DLBCL) are at an elevated mortality risk from non-cancer causes even after the disease is cured, according to a study published in *Cancer*. risk of death from factors other than this malignancy, including treatment-related side effects and disease-induced immunosuppression., blood disease ((highest risk), infection, gastrointestinal disease, vascular diseases, and lung disease between 0 and 59 months post-diagnosis were particularly high; after 59 months these risks were lower, though not non-existent.

I began my writing of this book January 2016 in Costa Rica where I sat in the shade listening to the crashing waves of the ocean, the squawking of the macaws and the howl of the howler monkeys. I began to let it all out, just let it flow, as I called it a brain dump. No direction just letting the computer capture it all. But getting there wasn't easy and I'm not talking just about the travel hurdles, even before that, just committing to go. You see, I really wanted to go from the day I saw it advertised, they needed a non-refundable deposit and then full payment a few months before the retreat. And then there were flights to get, but but but, what if what if what if I can't go. Will I be well to go; well by still being in remission and well enough to meet the demands of it-was I up to it mind and body. I had never been one that doubted or vacillated before this. If I saw something, wanted to do something, I would make a decision and go for it – simple as that, but now I was fearful of making ANY decisions, commitments; again, that what if, so just in case... It was a great trip, I spent a lot of time on the mat synthesizing emotions, sensations and crying. Never tears of sadness, but tears of gratitude that I could be in that beautiful place with wonderful people and just be Faith. The fact that I was there, wow, something that cannot be put into words.

And then I book a Trans Atlantic Cruise, solo, was what I called my liberation cruise. 2 weeks on a ship of strangers, and the transformations begin to happen. Drinking Prosecco every night with new friends, and then the dancing. The moving, the swaying, the shaking, the sweating, getting transfixed in the beat-Life, LIVING was happening. I got a chance to reconnect to being a living breathing me, and I felt liberated from that person who just a year before had the last 5 hr round of R-CHOP pumped in her veins. And it was a mere 2 weeks before the cruise I had the port taken out of my left chest wall. That was my one-year remission celebration. The thoughts, feelings, concerns flowed into the computer by day, I cried remembering, I cried wondering how I made it through day by day, and then I cried-how I survived. But at the end of the cruise I felt I had shed a layer, like a snake slithering out of its skin. I went in Faith, I have Lymphoma, I am in remission, the cancer still controls me; I guess wearing a badge of courage. The little voice, tho, kept ticking off time, one year and one month and counting. Almost like a stop watch counting down to the explosion.

More time, life, work, the usual stuff and another everything looks good. So back to Costa Rica, the ocean waves, the birds, the monkeys and the iguanas. More Cruises, But the real liberation comes each time I make a commitment for something in the future, no second guessing, no hesitation, I have been freed, the chains holding me back are finally unlocked. Living in the present, accepting me now, not fretting over the past and wasting time and energy on the future. In the Moment and Loving It. And I like me now, gray hair, wrinkles, achy joints and all-gives me character. I am liberated. I've been asked why I don't color my hair, and I answer, as much as I do not like the silver hair I am much more interested in having a strong fit active body and living in wellness.

The Chemo Chronicles (This is My Personal Journal & Facebook Posts)

December 19, 2014   My friend Howard Kahen of Radiology Associates West Pasco, came thru for me. After our back and forth with the biopsy someone felt uncomfortable doing it so to another option requiring an endoscope. Howard looked at the films said what's the big deal. Made room for me on the schedule and if all goes as planned on Monday morning success. The sooner we get results we can start what they call treatment. I have other words for it but I'll keep that to myself. I've had a big reality check in that this thing is gonna get me if I do nothing and still will despite "treatment" and the "treatment" can do me in but if I don't use weaponry that is available I don't have any chance. So, see you Monday Howard Kahen and thanx for being you.

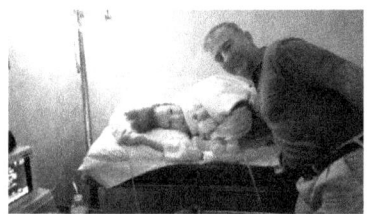

After the biopsy going in through my liver to grab a piece of the periportal node.   Had to lay on my side to put pressure to keep it from bleeding. No fun here. Thank you, My John and Carol, for being there with me. And thank you Mary Pigott, the nurse who joined my healing team.

December 24, 2014   Back home stress filled morning but at least we know the identity and have a plan. First pathology report showed a slow spleen-based lymphoma but in 3 weeks it has infiltrated my body acting as a totally different player. Also, I went from feeling great to not feeling great and knowing my body was being taken over by this invader. So today the REAL path report came in, large b cell very aggressive. So now I can get into warrior mode and direct my battle and meditation. I didn't want to wait another day to ignite the flame of victory in this battle so I start Friday 8:30 am to start the killing machine of those m.th.r f..k..rs. And since I am going to lose my hair to RCHOP I am going to get it cut short first. And yikes that dammed gray is going to show off so send good vibes. Show John the love and I'll keep posted as I can. So, for today and tomorrow John, Dock Dog, Karma and I are together. And next week my Nick Tumminello will come visit.
Thank you, Shawn and Angel from New Attitude Salon in Port Richey, giving me my new look on Christmas Eve. Angel called it my first brave step. So, if I'm going to be losing my hair I figured I'd start with getting it going on my terms first and then we'll modify as needed. And my Carol Tracht-Kader there at my side smiling love you girl.

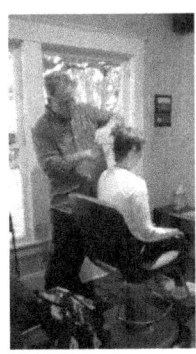

December 26, 2014   "As I arise this AM I contemplate contemplate contemplate. Did a brief warrior yoga practice reciting mantra for this journey. Want to enjoy my chai tea and just check in. Thank you to everyone for your love, healing energy, prayers and support. This is a journey of mind body & modern medicine. Gotta use what the technology brings but working to keep life in balance mind and body. I go into this today strong, focused, a fighter. A survivor and a victor. Today the eviction sign goes up and these cancer cells are told no more you are moving out and if you resist we're gonna crush you. So, I sign off for now til I can update. The warrior."

"Today I approach with dread, starting chemo feels worse than the diagnosis of a cancer. I realize now that all I have been and done is to prepare me for this. My strength, my focus, my meditation, and belief in inner strength and the universe. Please let me find that strength when I want to fill with tears. I am a Warrior; I am Strong; I am Focused; I am a Fighter; I am a Survivor; I am Victorious; I am Loved; I am blessed with so much. I leave my home to return forever changed. I leave with an invader inside of me taking over, and I return full of toxins. The work will then begin slowly eating away at the invader.

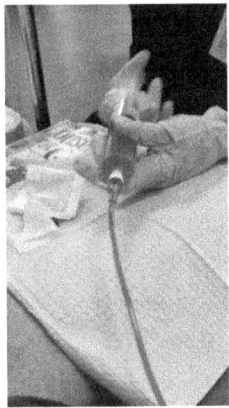

My mind and spirit will not be eaten. I am going to LIVE!"

December 27, 2014   24hrs post chemo, had a dystonic reaction to the nausea med; good thing I knew what it was because it was scary. But even worse it didn't help the nausea and vomiting either. I'm eating small quantities of food today and some things smell and taste foul. Basically, I feel like a toxic dump. But on the good side that highly toxic stuff put up the eviction notice for the cancer and I'm going to eradicate those invaders. Got some time on the mat a clear warm day so I did an easy practice by the water. And best of all downward dog was great that is my go to pose. Now coming back up that needs to move slow. So, one treatment down. We are on the path and need to be in the present and go with the flow. My bestie Carol Tracht-Kader came over to stay with me and cooked for me all day all good stuff. So we shall see what tomorrow will bring and I look forward to having my Nick Tumminello and Jaclyn Gough here for a few days next week.
I am surrounded by such love and my mat always welcomes me even at 4 am as it did this am. Nothing like a lavender eye pillow listening to Snatam Kaur and my body supported on the mat. Meditate move breathe, breathe some more and repeat.

January 3, 2015   Yesterday was exciting went out with my Mobile Medical Team partner Kim to see patients. Was good to feel productive and not see myself as a patient. But today I just feel weird. Don't know if it is the invader trying to stake claim, effects of the chemo or coming down off of 100 mg of prednisone a day for 5 days. For someone who didn't take meds/drugs I feel uncomfortable in my own body like a toxic dump and disconnected from what is causing what.
So glad I am in Florida as I put my mat out on our pool deck this am and got some time to breathe, move, reconnect and meditate. I am confident there is something I am supposed to learn here and hopefully share with others. I, with my focus and fight, try to stay in the present and in the flow and not divert from the positive

January 5, 2015   Went to Moffitt today for another opinion with the lymphoma specialist Dr. Sokol. Very interesting and good visit. I went with my friend Carol, a microbiologist and a stack of papers of research and presentations on lymphoma. We weren't going to let him off the hook. He answered all our questions was never condescending or rushed. I came out of the appointment feeling more positive than I have since getting the bad news. Gonna be a rough ride but I have the spirit to make this a win.
Cool thing just happened. I've been doing lots of research on lots of stuff and found a product called Healios that is used for chemo and radiation induced mucositis. At first my doc was skeptical but when he went to the website he saw formulated by an oncologist and research info. He gave me the go ahead to use it. In the meantime, I had contacted the company and received a call from them and an email from the doc himself. So, I was able to get them to send a case of product for them to share with patients who need it. Awesome. Www.healiosproducts.com/oncology. And they say it helps other causes of oral mucosal breakdown as well. And thank you Cindy my chemo nurse who is copying the research I brought in and making sure others are aware.

January 8, 2015   Friday, I go back to North Bay Hospital for a short procedure, to get my Infusaport in. This medical consumerism is getting far too regular. I am first on the list at 7:30 AM so gotta be there at 6. Hopefully I'll still be bleary eyed and sleepy and not noticing how hungry I am as I am starved as soon as I get up. Luckily my angel Patti McMurrian, RN, will be there as she rescheduled herself to be my pre-op nurse. And last spoke to my other angel Pat Dombrowski, RN, she said she was going to be there as she is post op. So, I know I am in good hands, it is a simple procedure and hopefully I'll be home by noon. I've been feeling good this week, rested, strong, good appetite. Next week on the 15th is round 2, let's get it on and keep the healing going. I can't thank everyone enough for all the love and support that has been sent my way. Wow, I am a blessed girl.

When I made the shift from Oh crap to what can I learn, what can I share and how I can embrace the journey for my growth I found the negative scary thoughts stuffed so far back as all the positives are so huge and prominent. Last night sitting on the couch with my John laughing and eating a Talenti Gelato bar I realized that at that moment I wasn't a cancer patient but a woman just enjoying the special things in life. And even better I'm teaching this am. So glad to be able to share some time on the mat with my Flow Yoga family.

January 9, 2015   All done, port is in. My angel Patty McMurrian RN was with me pre and post. No complications and nothing like versed, fentanyl and propofol. I remember nothing after I got on the surgery table til I woke up in post op. My wonderful John welcomed Me to come home bearing a chai latte. Eyes feel heavy hopefully this will clear as lots to do later today.

January 14, 2015   Hard to believe it is almost 3 weeks since I started my chemo journey. I have felt great the last week and a half, no side effects from the chemo other than hair falling out, lots of energy, appetite good, feeling strong and the few symptoms of the lymphoma have disappeared, the few nodes my probing fingers could find and the sweats have gone. So, I am very happy with the progress. Tomorrow I go for round 2, I am consistent on the mat, getting in some resistance work and trying to get out and do more walking. I've even been seeing patients. It is funny how I am almost eager to go for chemo tomorrow, as it will take me one more step closer to clearing my body of the invasion that seeks to take over. Having been a plant-based eater, organic as much as possible for over half my life, I know that just a healthy lifestyle, the right supplements, immune boosters etc. isn't all it takes. I go to the health food store to purchase my organic juices etc. and everyone is trying to sell me on a supplement/immune booster to fight the cancer and detox my body. I explain to them that if all that stuff was the answer I wouldn't be in this situation right now. Furthermore, the idea is not to detox from the horrible drugs that are being pumped in right now because you want them to be active and do the do. Will detox when the chemo is complete and resolution has been achieved. I have researched, discussed, questioned, and get a kick out of how everyone thinks they have the answer from something they've read etc. I even had a clerk in Whole Foods tell me I should stop chemo immediately to eat apple seeds and drink alkaline water - really. I admit that I haven't been consuming apple seeds but I've been eating an alkaline diet for years. (except of course from the occasional glass of wine -none now). I wish there was something better than the chemo as it is but we need to really understand and know all the info that is being thrown at us. There are no quick fixes or magic cures. So please keep sending your support as I continue on this journey. I expect by next week I'll be wigging, just ordered wig No. 2.

January 15, 2015   "Chemo round 2, today is embraced not with dread but with let's get it on. So many shifts, transformations and more for the better. So much to be grateful for. I have so much love and support surrounding me. I must admit it has surprised me. The last 2 weeks have been great. First Nick and Jackie came to visit for New Years and although I had a bit post chemo fatigue we had a wonderful family time. There were a couple of days with the prednisone I felt weirded out but otherwise all good. Got to teach, seeing patients, hair getting shorter and thinner, should be gone in a few days. So, all in all I've been feeling really good. They are trying another antiemetic in the mix and hope it helps. I also have essential oils and Queaze Ease. So round 2 knock out the bad guys and the Warrior is Victorious.

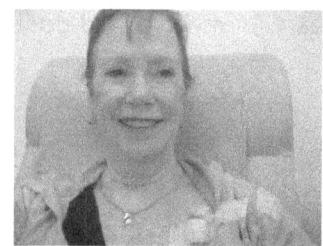Chemo 2/1st using the Infusaport, my alien implant.

January 16, 2015   Yesterday chemo round 2 was a big yay. First, I gained back 3 lbs., lab numbers are good. One value LDH goes up in cancers and one of the prognosticators is its level. Mine was elevated but not in the extreme and is now in a normal range yay, high is bad. This means the fuel that the cancer feeds on is being depleted ☺ for those of you who heard green tea is good for cancer one reason is it can lower LDH. Other counts are good and I'm feeling good. The added antiemetic, a small dose of Ativan and Queaze Ease an aroma therapy product for nausea, I am post chemo puke free, yay. Slept all nite and am now sipping my chai tea. Only downer is I have to use almond milk in it I do prefer the goat's milk but doesn't agree with me now.

It is really quite weird that when the cytotoxic drugs are being pumped in I can feel some of the nodes reacting. I equate this to an exterminator coming for a roach infestation and how they start running frantically to save themselves only to succumb once the poison takes over. Maybe being really in touch with your body also gives a little imagination too ☺ Well I am eating some wonderful lovingly mashed organic purple and sweet potatoes whipped up by my friend Carol for me and has fresh cinnamon in it.

Tired of clumps of hair falling out on the pillow at night going up my nose, getting so thin and bald spots so thank goodness my next-door neighbor wonderful friend Ingrid is a retired hairdresser with all the tools and my friend Carol was there to urge her on, I got buzzed. And I feel free. Sorry Shawn & Angel Nally (From New Attitude Hair Salon) that I had to let all the beautiful work go for now. But when it grows back in we will have lots of fun. So, John says I have a small head and Carol is going to call me Vin Diesel and I think he is pretty hot. Now we need to get some henna and get creative with the new canvas area. Shannon Jonas this made me think of you in Rishikesh, wish I had the Ganga to send my hair down as you did. Gotta keep smiling and having fun.

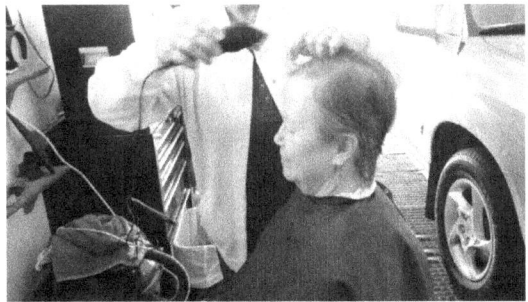 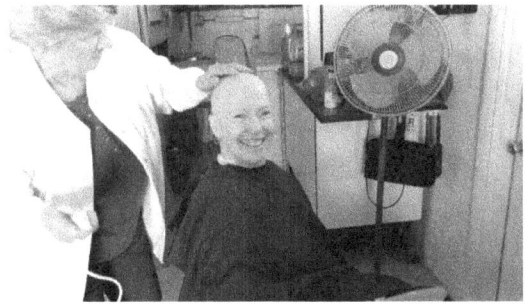

January 18, 2015   My wonderful son Nick is hanging out with me while John is on a business trip. It is so great having him here. Yesterday started the day off feeling pretty good and by afternoon was aching so bad. I received my Neulasta shot little after 4 on Friday, didn't have a reaction to it after my first treatment but wow, it was something. Suddenly mid shaft humerus and femur, my skull, mandible, sternum and pelvis couldn't be touched and my neck just stiffened up so bad. Was scary as I was afraid I was coming down with something bad. But turns out not an unusual reaction, so I'll be prepared next time, yikes. But all is well today, Nick and I took a nice walk, got some fresh air, chatted up all the while. So happy to have him here. And thank you Elaine Ning brought me her healing soothing delicious special food. And this great oil she massaged into my neck. Oh my.

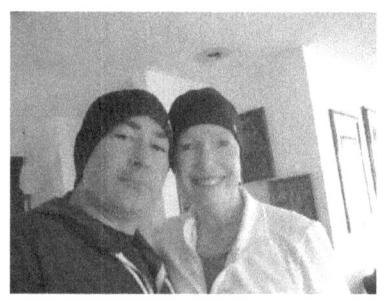

January 20, 2015   It has been so great having my baby boy here with me while John is out of town. He has been such great company and having him here has made me feel more safe and secure. This first week from chemo I am on a high dose of prednisone and it makes me feel shaky and weak, comes on suddenly without warning so I am uncomfortable driving and doing a lot until later in the afternoon when it seems to pass. I have figured out it isn't as bad if I take one 20 mg tablet at a time every hour times 5, rather than all at once, but then I may be feeling OK and suddenly, yikes. Nick's being here has worked for him as well as he is working on his second book and this has given him time to sit at the computer writing without the usual demands of being at home. It also gives me a chance to be a proud Momma when I introduce him to folks, when we do get out:-) And yesterday I went out for the first time with a wig, in fact wore one wig earlier in the day and wore a different one later. Still have eye brows (although they have always been thin) and eye lashes, so lots of mascara still works. I did buy some false eye lashes just in case but haven't cracked them out yet. So, all is well, I will miss Nick when he leaves tonite. Even in this time of unknown, not being at my best, I feel so grateful for all I have. I am surrounded by so much love and support, I am very blessed.

January 21, 2015   Been up since 4:30 am. Took last of the 100 mg of prednisone yesterday so today totally wigged out. Palpitations, can't concentrate or stay on task, even typing this out is challenging, lips are tingling. Fed Dock Dog at 6 am and can't even get myself together to get him out. Can't believe it is 9:15 and I'm still spinning my wheels. But as long as these drugs are doing their job I can handle it. Good news I should be functional if not tomorrow then Friday so I'll get productive again. Wow.

January 23, 2015   Love this. Definitely what I spend time thinking about these days. Lessons to learn, hurdles to rise above and finding the essence of living in everything, everyone and every moment. Each day has a unique flavor and some are flavors I don't like (I do miss my dark chocolate) but I am thrilled to have the experience. My John went back into work today after spending his first day home fixing a plumbing problem. I played on the couch all day yesterday as I had no energy and then slept from 9 pm til 7 this morning. Today I should be able to get out of the house as I'm now on day 3 of no prednisone so hopefully getting somewhat back in balance. When I had patients tell me how they hated being put on steroids I would wonder just how bad could it be. So, I am certainly empathetic to that now. Yikes.

January 25, 2015   This is beautiful, John and I had our first day together yesterday, I mean together being, doing; we went out for a nice long walk. It was cool, breezy, but clear; we walked where we hadn't been for years to Brasher Park and enjoyed life together. The waves were really kicking up (our standard) as we stopped and embraced in the warmest longest speechless hug ever. We walked back home, ran a few errands, had a bite to eat and all the while smiling at one another, laughing and holding hands. I thanked him for the wonderful walk and he said how much he enjoyed it and asked if we could do it again today and let's go somewhere special and make it an outing. Wow. So, as I ponder all that has been and will be and as I read about the mind body connection in cancer. I don't relate to what is written about regret, resentment and anger. I felt before all this blessed, loving and peaceful, but maybe something in that hug, in taking the time now that those little moments the small things ARE bigger and more important and should come first. I admit to always trying to get everything done first before giving myself the time to just enjoy but I now realize I had it backwards. So, I open for what this illness is to teach me. I am learning every day.

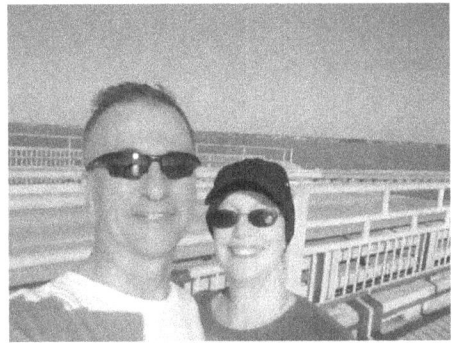

February 5, 2015   Here I am extermination #3 in progress. My third gratitude is about rediscovery. I was a runner for MANY years, in fact my life revolved around running in so many ways. Going out feeling and hearing the earth and sometimes snow beneath my feet. Breathing deeply the earth's prana. Listening to the rustle of life from the little creatures scurrying around. The essence of feeling fully present ALIVE and connected to the universe. And when I had to let running go because the discomfort in the hip and knee became more than the joy, I grieved. But now I have found that connection again. No, I haven't started running; wouldn't be too smart right now. But taking long walks, breathing deeply, listening, feeling, noticing, feeling totally ALIVE, living it's back. So, I am grateful I am taking the time for me not putting everything and everyone else first. I am allowing myself to live for me. And I hope it makes me a better wife, mother, friend, teacher, and PA, as I once again really enjoy the little things. Thanks for listening.

February 11, 2015   Yesterday was day 5 of 100 mg prednisone and like the previous times it is definitely accumulative in affecting sleep. No sleep at all last nite, the 2 nites before I was up at 4. Yikes. My insides jumping around, lips numb but the good news is today being crash day off of them, so sleep is in my immediate future, tonite...... Still so grateful not to have a lot of the other problems with chemo, no nausea, appetite is good, in fact on the steroids when I get that wave of extreme hunger I'll eat anything that doesn't run away from me. As long as I don't need to cut it cause the shakes makes using a knife dangerous. On the up side, after today I have 2 good weeks ahead of me til Extermination #4. And even better, I am scheduled to sub some classes, the next 2 Sundays and Tues next week. Doesn't get better than that being back on the mat at Flow.

February 13, 2015   Yikes today was supposed to be bounce back day and it isn't. Developed pain on my right side last night that hasn't resolved. Still have some shakes and appetite is missing. Have a fever, getting iv fluids, vitals not right. I feel weak and will be going for a chest x-ray and going on antibiotics. And I've been doing so good. Bummer. Just a little detour where the GPS says recalculating.

February 14, 2015   Bad day, fevers continue, pain continues, Doc is putting me in the hospital. I am really scared.   Now I know why I was feeling so bad. I have a blood clot in my lung with a pneumonia. Hi ho hi ho not quite the way I wanted to go but knew something was wrong and pulmonary embolus was high on my list of most likely.

February 16, 2015   I am breaking out of this joint. Yay. Was a big to do cause one of the meds is injected but I found it at one of the pharmacies I deal with and it is questionable if the insurance will cover it so, he has offered a nice cash price. I so want to go. All vitals perfect for 24 hrs. and I've been free of the pain that brought me in for 24 hrs. so I'm psyched and ready. Feel good and antsy. Not thrilled to be on blood thinners and antibiotics and certainly not thrilled to have a PE and pneumonia but thrilled that my body made a prompt come back. Yay

February 17, 2015, I awoke this morning in a state of complete Bliss. In my cozy bed actually slept wow amazing.

 I got the coolest videos from my YogaFit Training Systems Worldwide friends. I don't have the technology to share the actual videos, but I want to thank Beth Shaw, Shaye Molendyke, Sandi Cartwright, Kristy Morton Manuel, Jenny Baldwin, Jennifer Mumford, Kenny, and the mastermind LaMor Silas. When I watched them, I had the biggest smile on my face and tears streaming down my face. Love you guys and I can't wait to be back with you all. Here are the lyrics, I am so blessed.

"Faith" by George Michael (lyrics personalized for our friend Faith)!

Well, we know it would be nice
If we could heal your body
We know not everybody
Has got a body like you.
Ah..., no thinking twice
Before we give our hearts away
We know the games cancer plays
And we want to stop it, too.
Bet .. you need some time off ... from the emotion,
Time to pick your heart up off the floor.
And when you feel the love from our devotion,
Well, it takes a strong woman, but our Faith
Will show it the door,
'Coz we gotta have Faith
We gotta have... Faith
Yes, We've gotta have Faith, Faith, Faith
We gotta have Faith, Faith, Faith.
Lady, we're wanting your cancer to go away
Saying please, please, please go away
You say its giving you the blues.
Please know we mean every word we say
Can't help but try to brighten up your day
And wish it would go away too!
Before this river becomes an ocean
Before you make fun of our silly video
Oh lady, its not a foolish silly notion
We want you to be well and back with us at MBFs and more ...
Coz We gotta have Faith...
(repeat chorus)
LaMor

<u>February 20, 2015</u>   Wednesday the oncologist switched me from Coumadin for my PE to Xarelto. Even though I was taking the Coumadin same time every day and I was avoiding the highest Vit K foods the numbers were going down instead of up to the targeted level. I explained to the oncologist that when you put a vegetarian on Coumadin the only way you will achieve target is thru starvation as almost all vegetables contain vitamin K so just not eating spinach and kale isn't going to cut it. So yesterday I unashamedly made myself a sandwich with homemade humus, gluten free bread and lots of steamed spinach, yum yum. Last night I steamed up broccoli, cauliflower, cabbage, onions, all the Vit K rich foods, heaven. I feel like a punching bag, get a punch to the jaw go down and hover just above the ground suddenly popping back up with a smile

on my face, repeat. As long as I keep getting up with a smile.............. Still have the lung pain but nothing like that that drove me to the hospital, have to admit the pain was the worst I have ever experienced like someone stabbing me repeatedly and then twisting the knife. Yikes. But today I am going to see patients, and I am looking forward to Sunday when I am going to sub the 10 am class, and then again Tuesday at 10 am. I feel like I lost almost an entire week, last Friday was supposed to be bounce back day, I did get to take a nice walk yesterday not fast but very enjoyable, so hope to do more this weekend and try to strengthen myself up for extermination #4 on Thursday. This is a crucial one as they will repeat the PET scan after this one to see if there has been clearing of the lymphoma, they look for the metabolic activity in the lymph nodes. Or I shall say hoping to not see any metabolic activity in them. So still smiling, going with the Flow and counting my blessings.

February 24, 2015   My wonderful friend Kevin Witt drove over here this afternoon in the rain to bring me a root bake. I just heated it up and had some for dinner, delicious. All good stuff. He never leaves my John out as he brought him fresh baked banana bread. Such good friends. I'm so blessed and grateful.

February 26, 2015   Am just now finishing my 4th extermination process. This one is truth or dare as I will get a PET scan in 2 weeks to see how it is working. I've been anxious about it and wouldn't you believe I've slept the last 2 hrs. As I've been on this journey I've been trying to uncover its meaning but I don't relate to suggestions of pent up anger, resentment, disappointment, etc. But I saw a Facebook post with a picture of a flower and the word Be. And I began to cry because it is for me to simply be. This is my challenge as I cannot affect, expedite, or change; just need to BE, wow. So, my gratitude is for everything that is. So, I can simply BE. Wow. Headed home how totally uneventful this one was.

February 27, 2015   This is what I am challenged with right now, being a patient patient. It will be 3 weeks before I know results of how the chemo is working, I can't help but have concern and fear. Even my oncologist said he would have the same if he were in my place. I am so grateful to everyone who has been supporting me on this journey, and I look at each day as a gift. I think this is even a little more challenging than the initial diagnosis and moving forward with treatment, feeling empowered with using the tools available. But this is a waiting game right now, nothing to do but to Be.

Here it is I finally found it. It's been 2 days since I saw this, I began to cry and then it was gone. I immediately knew this is what the meaning of all this is. As I've meditated, moved, questioned and sought what it is I am to learn from this journey, I am continually left still with "what?" I feel blessed with my life, not that things have always been rosy but everything has aligned itself to bring me to a positive place. I've grown, I've explored, I've learned, I've transformed and evolved. And even before my diagnosis I've felt and expressed gratitude, I am surrounded with love and try to keep what doesn't serve me in the past, even if something is happening today not to bring to the future but to let it go, make it history. As I spoke to my son Nick Tumminello and my friend Kimberly Brust the other day, 2 very get it done successful folks I shared how this journey has been so challenging and not in how it has changed my daily activities, putting chemical poisons in my body and getting radiation, all things that I have spent sooooo many years avoiding, and knowing that my body which has always been so strong, resilient and so quick to heal has become the enemy imprisoning me, unable to see beyond the prison boundaries. It is that what has made me successful in life, being able to do what needs to be done and find ways around and to overcome obstacles, that in this situation other than keeping my mind and body as strong, calm and focused as I can, I cannot affect how the chemo does its work. I can't change the genetic makeup of this lymphoma, I can't affect its ability to be challenged and overridden by the chemo or its ability to become resistant with its own goal of survival. Perhaps it is my medical training, too much knowledge here and I read read read and then read more, trying to seek more insight and understanding because I know I certainly can't direct or control. In many cases I wish I were ignorant to the facts, that I could just have blind trust. So, when I saw this, this is it. I shared this with my friend Angel Nally as I knew she would get it. And she pointed out to me a very old, grand tree that has weathered all kinds of storms, is overgrown by moss and vines, has some broken limbs, and she asked me what does the tree do with all this. And I said just "Be".

March 3, 2015   Wow, what a difference having some sleep makes. I broke down and took a gentle pharmacologic (was prescribed and sits in the cabinet) with a melatonin and I slept. So last day of this cycle, the 100 mg prednisone but at least I feel I have some more strength to cope that I got some rest. Yayyyyyyy Maybe I can even get something done today.

March 5, 2015   Last night stepped out to get comfortable with being uncomfortable. As a medical practitioner I am accustomed to not just listening to others troubles but to always put my needs aside as my patients come first. I have done the same with Flow Yoga and all the wonderful folks that spend their time and energy there. Being at what I call "truth or dare" getting my PET scan next week and then the results, I admit that I am finding myself feeling a bit more apprehension than I have during this course as I felt strong in that I was doing EVERYTHING I could to handle this course. But now it is not just directed towards treatment but is the treatment doing everything it should be doing. I went to a support group and so glad I did. Met some wonderful people and sharing highs, lows, concerns, smiles and laughter was great. I shared with them about learning to just "Be" as I feel that is my biggest challenge right now. Always being the one to get something done and make it successful, just being, wow. Came off the steroids yesterday, slept 8 hrs. unaided, so today is going to be a great day.

March 9, 2015   This week is a week I have looked forward to eagerly and with anxiety. My journey into medical consumerism began 4 months ago, wow, and with my recently completing my fourth round of chemotherapy it is time to assess the effectiveness with a PET scan tomorrow morning. I'll have the results on Friday. At first, I focused on handling chemo side effects, and was quite impressed that I had few negative side effects and was functioning very well. Over the last week I have not felt well, maybe accumulated effects of chemo but of course my mind will travel to the more ominous negative reasons. Got to admit this is the most challenging experience, and glad I get some temporary relief going out walking, being in nature definitely makes me feel better, and spending time on the mat. But unfortunately, not feeling well is making this a bigger challenge right now. For someone that has always been strong and able to steer most situations to the positive, it is very unsettling knowing there is nothing I can do but "Just Be". I bring the photo of the flower into my mind, breathe into it and try to find some peace if just for the short time. So, Friday will be the day, and happily my son Nick and Jaclyn will be here on Sunday to spend a few days. So, if the last 4 months have gone quickly I am sure this week will do so too.

I have tears of joy. My PET scan is CLEAR. There is no evidence of the hyper metabolic lymph nodes indicative of active lymphoma. It appears the word remission is possibly in my future. 2 more treatments and then follow ups. Need to start planning life. Thank you everyone for all your love, support, prayers and healing energy.

March 21, 2015   Had a great double Gong Immersion last nite. Thank you Rae Clauser and Mary Ann, your intention of new beginnings was PERFECT. Gotta share that during the gong I could feel the energy vibrating through my body in waves, emotional, clearing, joyful waves. A feeling of connection within my body, mind and spirit and the energy around me. Many times, during the gong I felt a smile come across my lips that radiated into my heart. It was a connection to my restored wellbeing and hopes for the future.

This is a complete contrast to the gong of Dec before my correct diagnosis and an assumption based on the initial pathology report that all was well. It was during the gong that I felt like a brick wall no matter how much I tried to invite the vibration into my body it bounced off, the harder I tried to invite it, accept it the more it resisted. The only time the vibration was accepted is if I brought the thought of being loved into my mind. Tears filled my eyes and down my face and I knew something was terribly wrong. But it did affirm LOVE.

I know we can't quantify or qualify these experiences, but I know all the love, prayers, support, and healing energy that has been shared with me has increased the effectiveness of the modern medicine. I am so grateful, and thankful, it is spring, I have a new beginning, wow. Didn't look like this in Dec. Thank all of you again for being with me encouraging me along on this journey.

March 22, 2015   My husband just said I appear discombobulated (however that is spelled). And all I could think was no shit. Day 4 of 100 mg prednisone. 2 more days to go. And then one more round in April, I can do it. I've got the good stuff going, healing, moving on with life, all good. And then he gave me a big loving hug, I needed that.

March 24, 2015   How crazy I am now looking for medical information on Google. A week after my fourth treatment I began having some intermittent vocal changes, a hoarseness that would come and go, no pain or any sense of discomfort just loss of volume with a gravely sound. And since it was the time I was anxious about the upcoming PET scan, results and knowing where my life was headed I attributed it to stress. I also thought about my throat chakra and how during this time I feel like my expression has been stifled. My voice loss has now progressed to decreased volume, roughness and just a sense of feeling like my vocal cords aren't working as opposed to what we have all experienced with that thick feeling when having a cold or just a strained voice. My oncologist doesn't seem concerned but also doesn't say much about it, just says if it doesn't clear to see an ENT. Well of course I'm not just sitting here so hi ho hi ho to Google we go. And there are lots of others blogging same thing. And all say that their oncologist acts like they've never heard it before. So, I am going to see an ENT, in fact looking for a voice specialist, but all along I've thought it was the chemo. Hey, after all, I spent years teaching aerobics in gymnasiums yelling and frequently having hoarseness and then years later getting intermittent hoarseness when teaching too many classes even when using a microphone, so I expect it is just going to a place of weakness. But what is that about that the pro's act like they've never heard about it before. Yikes. So, if anyone has any info on this please send it my way, and if you are in the Tampa area (Pasco/Hernando/Pinellas/Hillsborough) do you know of any good ENT/Laryngologist that you recommend. Guess this is a time I really need to start listening more - another lesson for me on this journey. If this is the worst of the side effects, I am still way ahead of the curve.

Found this on the Web today: www.cosmopolitan.com

<u>8 Things Not to Say to Someone Who Has Cancer</u>

Just saw this and had to share. OMG, they say cancer changes you in ways other than the disease, hell yes. But how do you begin to explain it. it changes daily from the thoughts of yikes, to yay, to will there be next year to why the hell not. And I know it is hard for the friends and family as well. So thought this was really good.---
http://www.cosmopolitan.com/health-fitness/a38100/things-not-to-say-to-someone-with-cancer/
And an FYI, I did have someone ask me my prognosis, I would definitely say that is a no no. They've never called me back.

<u>April 8, 2015</u>   Today I got to experience a totally different emotion on my medical consumer journey, wow, this has been an experience. Up until Nov I hadn't had a doctor, didn't need one, healthy, clean diet and lifestyle. No risk factors, so no need, so that means the only practitioner patient relationships I had was as being the practitioner. So today I saw my hematologist/oncologist Dr. Uday Dandamudi, he was the first person I saw when I was in the hospital for the Great Spleen Adventure and he has seen me through guiding my care to remission. Tomorrow is my last chemo, #6 Extermination. I asked for a photo and we departed with him saying I'll see you in 3 weeks just to do blood work and check on you, and when I went to schedule they said he wasn't going to be there after April 22. OMG, like stab me in the heart, I can't believe the sense of abandonment, wow. When I reflect on when I got the pathology in December and thinking my only planning was leaving this wonderful life and now I am planning on going to a Yoga Training and an Alaska cruise, I have him to thank, and have to admit I not only am grateful to him but have a feeling of dependence. I trust him, respect him, and really like him as a person. I am so grateful for him. And yes, I do have an opportunity to follow him, I have a good idea where he is going, but the Florida Cancer Affiliates have been really good to me. They have helped me where my insurance didn't cover, I go to support group there and have gotten to know everyone, so there is a comfort level and I am really grateful to them as well. But I do understand he has to take care of himself and his family. Yikes. Wow, this medical consumerism really sucks.

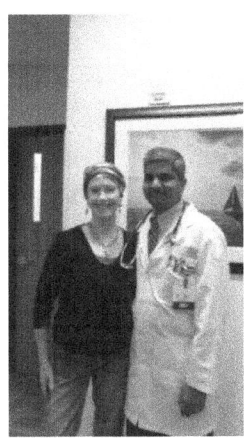

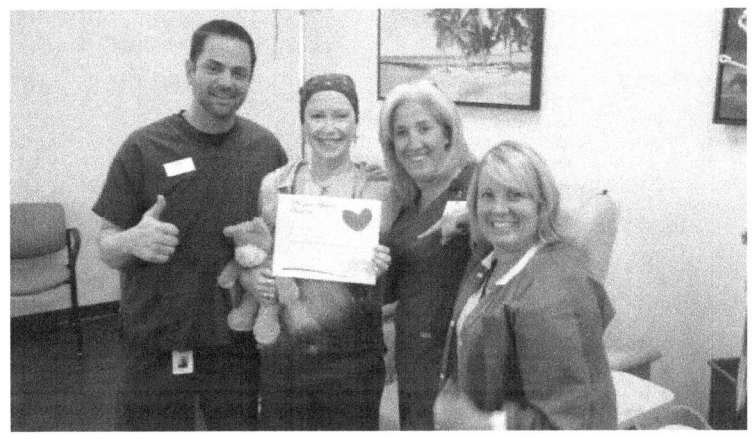

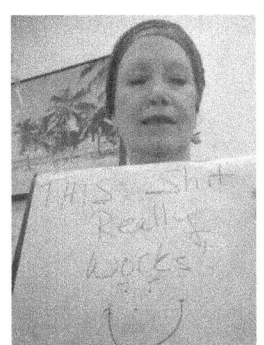

April 9, 2015   I am done. Started off amazing Bunnie McCormack came over and did Reiki on me then Carol Tracht-Kader picked me up went to the studio and I taught the 10 am class. She then dropped me off at chemo I ran into Nancy Britton who works for Florida Cancer affiliates. During my chemo I chatted with a very nice woman on my right and when she left a very nice woman took the chair to my left. We then chatted about stuff. Got her turned on to Helios which helps with the oral breakdown and they had the product to give to her. And we discussed sleep problems options and she asked her doctor and got a script. So, time went quickly. How cute they give this certificate. But yayyyyyy I'm done. Funny I taught Tues nite at Flow and I commented how I felt like nothing was wrong and Liz Dono reminded me nothing is wrong.

April 10, 2015   I talk to myself, many times out loud and then others silently to myself. I have emphasized in the present the effectiveness of my treatments, (sometimes even yelling - "the chemo is kicking your ass cancer" the healing that is happening, and the reclamation of my body, life and well-being. Even when I'm getting Reiki I am saying to myself healing energy. I do think it really makes a difference as people see me, it is obvious I'm on chemo as I am a baldy, almost no eyelashes or brows either, but they frequently comment (even strangers) how healthy I look. And I am sure it isn't just yoga, walking, healthy eating, it is what I am feeding my mind.

April 12, 2015   Here I am reminding myself I can make it thru, this is the last time 100 mg prednisone crazies. I stuff myself silly like I haven't eaten in forever. I flit from one thing to another, can't concentrate, unroll my yoga mat and even find that not being comfortable. I know it is temporary, always is, but it is just so weird to be so uncomfortable in my own body. Just this damn drug, but gotta say since it is part of the chemo regime that has brought me into remission it can't be that bad. 3 days and counting and it is crash day. From there I will start to shake the chemo side effects while hoping to keep all the good effects, looking forward to weight training again (was to no avail while on chemo, can't build while the cells are on stop), getting back to teaching on a regular basis, continuing with long walks, and now I am planning lots of good stuff. Time with yoga friends in June, a special vacation in July with family and friends, and looking forward to being able to eat lots of different foods. While on chemo you are supposed to avoid anything raw because of the chances of bacteria, how I am eager to bite into a strawberry and feel the crunch of a stick of celery. Oh my. And salad, can you imagine I haven't had a salad since the end of December. Not sure when the immune system starts to rev up but I can assure you when I get the it should be OK, a celery stick with hummus is going to be my first indulgence.

April 18, 2015   Went out today sporting the baldness, as it was in the 80's, humid and our Florida sun is already hot and beating down. I went to Whole Foods, and only there would a 62-year-old bald woman get a compliment on her earrings from the probably 18 yr. old male checkout clerk. But the earrings are rockin, made by Carol Tracht-Kader and without hair nothing to conceal them. Also, I went into my stash of long forgotten cosmetics and found cake eyeliner, much easier on the lids as now I have no lashes so lining away. But even hairless I am not going out without my makeup and jewelry. If I do you know we are in trouble.

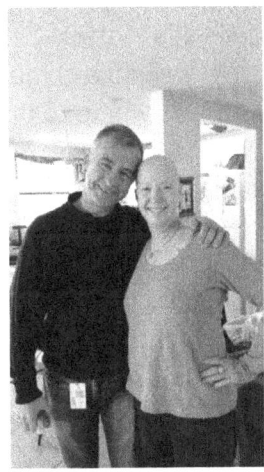

April 19, 2015   What a wonderful Sunday. Got a chance to teach this am, first class since getting the last chemo I was thinking it was going to be iffy all week but felt OK this am and what a wonderful group in our Sunday classes. The voice is still weak and scratchy so the microphone was soooo helpful. Thank you everyone for your support and being there. We had a special visitor, Elena from Milan. She was John's host on his work trips to Milan. Elena joined us on the mat for her first ever yoga class and then joined us for brunch. John did his killer goat cheese and spinach omelet. It was a little windy but not too windy for us to sit on the lanai, and the rain held out for us as well. She got the Florida experience on the water with an ibis in the yard. Great visit, great class, life is good.

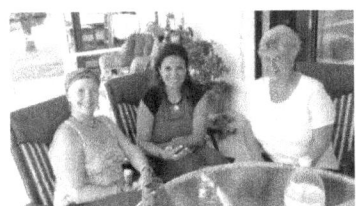

April 22, 2015   Did my after last treatment follow up with the Moffit lymphoma specialist Dr Sokol. I saw him after my first treatment, he agreed with everything that was being done at FL Cancer Affiliates led by my man Dr. Dandamudi. He had said then see you after the last treatment so today was the day. He commented how well I responded to the treatment and that is the BEST prognosticator. So good stuff, see him if I need him, and I can't wait til I can eat sushi. So happy times, good times, and eager to get some hair. But I owe it to Dr. D, he saved my life.

April 28, 2015   I am bummed and grateful. Received a phone call from Dr. Sokol the lymphoma specialist at Moffitt, after my visit last week he dove deeper into my chart and has some concerns about the aggressive nature of the lymphoma and its genetic markers, even though my PET scan is clear and symptomatically I'm doing well, he is concerned there can be small cells in my brain and he is proposing we do a prophylactic "intrathecal" chemo. In other words, they will do a spinal tap and put chemo in there.   There will be only 4 treatments one week apart and he wants to do it as soon as possible. The only issue is I am on a blood thinner Xarelto for my PE, gotta get off of that and get a plan going. Yikes. This is scary and I was so thrilled to be done with chemo, but I'm grateful he didn't let things go, he is the specialist and he is the only person I've heard mention this. Yikes, but at least he is talking prophylaxis not to treat, and we don't know if there are those small buggers there or not. Would only know if they start to do their thing and that would be bad. But shouldn't affect any of my upcoming plans so yay for that.

May 5, 2015   What a crazy week it has been. Last week was told I needed Intrathecal Chemo but I am not able to get it as I would need to be off of anticoagulants for a full month and with an unresolved pulmonary embolus and platelets elevated twice over the normal range, it is too risky. So, after speaking to my former oncologist who I trust, respect and really feel is up with everything, he didn't feel there was enough of an overwhelming indication for the procedure to stop the anticoagulant, when I went to see my new oncologist she didn't feel the procedure was definitely indicated in her opinion and felt that stopping the anticoagulants posed a more immediate risk. So, I am not going to get the procedure as you need to be off anticoagulants 7 days prior to the procedure and it would be 4 one week apart. So, I have to put that aside and go with the present flow. I am moving on with getting my life going again, getting stronger and feeling better every day. Was able to enjoy in Nick Tumminello's receipt of his award PT Trainer of the Year in Orlando.

June 21, 2015   Thank you everyone for bringing such great energy to Green Key Beach for our 108 sun salutations to honor the first International Day of Yoga and the Summer Solstice. Anyone who took photos please post them. For obvious reasons I wasn't able to take photos-I led the 108- yay. Who would have thought.

June 23, 2015   This is my first travel since my medical adventure began, you would have thought I had never flown before, my heart was racing, forgot to check in 24 hrs. beforehand (flying Southwest) so I am in C group. Oh well, happy to be here. Wiped the seat, belt and tray down with essential oils, not neurotic about germs but this is my first germ incubator being stuck in without being able to get away for a long time. I am just now not freaking if someone sneezes or coughs or not afraid to touch a menu.   Really if a menu touched the silverware I got phobic.   As the plane began to taxi down the runway I checked in as I always had being aware of when the tires leave the runway. But this time as I said to myself fly baby fly (as I always do when I fly) I began to cry. As this time, it wasn't just the plane flying but it was me spreading my wings again, taking off to new adventures and opportunity.

It cracks me up, I am getting compliments on my hair cut. Cut hell, it is a hair grow with silver spikes. What is that about!!!! One woman in the airport said "girl - you rock that hair " ha. So since I have no choice about the head, I want to have hair that is part Judy Dench, the "stop the insanity" of Susan Powter and Sinead O'Connor. Now that's rockin.

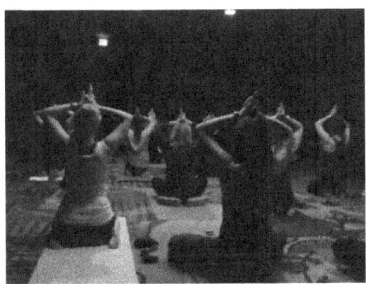 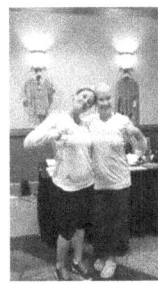

June 29, 2015

Had the most amazing 4 days in Minneapolis at YogaFit MBF. Was a time to reconnect with such great friends, to love on one another. But was so special for me as I was able to reconnect to myself. I have had 3 very transformational events at YogaFit MBF's and 2 with Beth Shaw leading the class. I recall a class in Sunny Isles, Fl when Beth turned off the air conditioner and opened the doors to the outside. The warm ocean air came in, sun illuminating the room - it was liberation and my tears flowed with my breath and sweat. Saturday in a darkened hotel room while hearing "something's happening here" my tears flowed as my being came together. The tightness I was holding in my hips melted away and my body moved without restraint. I felt healthy, happy and whole. Thank you to everyone for all the love and support I felt. Yoga is love, it is healing, it is living.

July 2, 2015   am living with this unrelenting stalker. It is hiding right now but like most stalkers can show up again at anytime and anywhere. I am embracing my gray hair, as I do have hair to show off now. So, life is good. And I am happy with waking up every day to see the sun, feel the breeze, the smile on my husband's face and feel his embrace, to hear all the good stuff with my son and friends. Breathe and flow on the mat alone and with others, And to just BE.

August 23, 2015 The 'Muscle of the Soul' may be Triggering Your Fear and Anxiety

www.themindunleashed.org

having done the Warrior training and being tapped into this, I experienced it firsthand. After my chemo ended I developed pain and constriction, FEAR. Psoas Psoas Psoas, classic. So even knowing doesn't mean you don't experience the problem but at least I now have strategies and knowledge for it.

August 24, 2015

New Yoga Walk-in Clinic Will Dole Out Yoga 'Prescriptions'

www.yogadork.com

This came at an appropriate morning. I am posed with a decision and this weekend helped me make it. I have been given a very good job offer but I have been concerned about being able to meet the demands put on me by the business. This is unusual for me as I am a not just get it done person but get more business and make it grow person. But since my cancer/chemo journey I don't always feel great with different aches, am often sleep challenged and just don't have the endurance I used to have. I have been quite confused over whether it is fear and anxiety or truly just the "new normal" and being in touch with it. So thurs I taught the morning and evening class at Flow Yoga/Pilates & Personal Training, Friday I was achy and could feel it. Sat I had a good day working in the yard, but the night was a fitful sleep and Sunday I lost my steam midafternoon. Although I still got work done at the studio moving equipment, furniture cleaning etc., I felt pretty drained. So, expecting to be able to sleep I was met with "not going to sleep tonite". So drastic measures were taken to get sleep and now I have the drug "hang over". This is the new reality and I think it is probably too early to take this job, as I would have to be on their time schedule and needs. Just not sure I can meet the demand right now. I think I am going to have to decline the opportunity right now, and who knows what the future will bring. And then I saw this about the Yoga Clinic. I keep saying I've had this experience and I need to do something to share it and help others. Cool!!!!!!!

August 26, 2015 Just had a wonderful 90 min outing with my John in Starkey park. It was a walking outing but I was able to jog 1/2 mile. Now did it 1/4 then walked and then another 1/4 but I'll take it. One step at a time reclaiming my health wellness vitality and LIFE. I am say yahoo for me.

My dear friend LaMor did a post that conjured up so much emotion. Wow, what a difference 4 years makes. At that time, I was on an adventure to Palm Springs to learn, experience and enjoy. Always looking for cool places to go, great people to meet (and have I ever) and how I can use what I learn and share. I would plan classes, events, work, travel etc. But I never knew the lessons would be used by me in a fight for my life. How life changed from going here and there to will I be around and if I see the sunrise the next day how will I feel. But I am grateful of the support from all my friends, and training with the tools that I would need and still do day to day, and to have learned to let go of judgment and attachment to embark on a journey that went against my beliefs. I thank Dr. Uday Dandamudi for having the confidence in me and being who he is so I could have the confidence in him to follow the path. I look at photos and want the old Faith back, but yet I embrace she is gone, there is the new Faith, stronger in many ways, wiser in many ways, and hopefully more patient, grateful, giving and kind. I smile under the silver streaks because I am truly blessed, grateful and ALIVE, living life. At times my mind wanders wondering if the alarm is going to sound ending this great renewal/remission or has the clock been turned off and I can just go about living not knowing as life was before. But it is you, my friends and family, who make life, it is living in this beautiful moment.

August 28, 2015 To all my wonderful friends who over this past year have kept me smiling, gave me the courage to go on, and the hope that it was all worth it. Thank you, it was worth it. Love you my friends.

August 29, 2015 Got out on the water in our kayaks before the rain. The water was calm a gentle breeze, was cloudy, not hot and we paddled up the river. On our way back heard a few thunder boomers and figured we needed to get back home. Paddled hard and strong, I counted 250 strong steady strokes without stop before I got to our dock. Felt good. Had some time to get in and showered up before the lightning and the rain. It is now pouring, and I have to tell you John stated it isn't going to rain, so watch out if he says that you can bet there is going to be a storm. Hadn't paddled since before I got sick, Nov 2014, yikes that long ago. So, this was exciting but also sad, because Dock Dog would watch us leave the dock and go out into the bayou and then bark in excitement to herald our return. All was quiet, no greeting, the house is so empty. We have Karma Kat but she could care!!!!! And secretly she is probably celebrating she doesn't have to share the house with a canine, he wanted to always say hi how ya doing? And she would look at him and go "really". The funny thing is, when we moved here we were warned to not let Dock go into the bayou off the boat dock as there are otters that would drown dogs, and we NEVER saw one, Dock had a sandy spot he would wade out into the water and hang out without event, but still never saw an otter. When we got back from our paddle John was doing something on the sea wall and guess what, an otter popped up right under his face and then it was gone. Weird.

9/9/2015 Here I am 5 months to the day since the last chemotherapy. I would have hoped I would be in a much better place physically and mentally now but it isn't better just different. I now have hair, silver short and allowing a little style to come into it, I like that. I am accustomed to looking at that me now and am OK with it as I am alive, and the old me is gone, this is the new me, although not the improved. I have described having cancer as a "mind fuck", it not only fucks with you, in every thought and action, but I feel my mind is fucked. Fear was never a constant companion of mine, in fact fear would only be a short-lived sensation when positioned in a dangerous or scary place or situation. But now I am Overwhelmed by it. Body tension, right psoas tightness and tenderness, insomnia, headaches, and is it just my mind or my body. The LDH is rising, that is a lymphoma marker, it was high when I was diagnosed and its elevation is a factor in staging. The oncologist states the other blood indices are good so he isn't so concerned with the LDH right now. Well, he doesn't have to worry, as I am doing the worrying for EVERYONE. A PET scan is scheduled in 2 weeks which will show if there is any lymph node activity and I monitor myself all day long, checking to see if I feel feverish, checking for any masses, nodes, since I don't sleep well I am now having to take a benzodiazepine to help me sleep. And because of that I feel hung over, tired, so I fret whether I have fatigue, a hallmark of lymphoma, or is it poor sleep and a benzo drugging and hang over. Yikes, I am depressed, but am I depressed causing neurosis, hyper vigilance, insomnia and fatigue or is it physical, the real deal and I am depressed because my inner self knows. All I can say is SHIT. I feel alive, "normal" on the mat teaching a class, transformed, calm and safe. Trying to just live, I am so grateful for having been given this extended time but I feel like I am living in a cruel joke. Remission, but knowing that it can be taken away at any time. It is that unknown, having no grounding right now that is the hardest. Sept 25 I will have the PET result, I keep telling myself to stop checking, just breathe, just be, the test will tell, no reason to do anything right now than just breathe.

9/14 Had some brief relief from the insomnia, taking melatonin, magnesium and .5 mg Ativan every evening around 8. falling asleep and sleeping til the morning. but suddenly awakening 2 am then 4 am and now on second night of not being able to fall asleep. So, here I am at 12:15 am, John is snoring away and I am writing. The sleep deprivation headache is building, the frustration is building and only leads to my mind running, worrying and fretting. There is a suicide bomber living inside of me, stalking and taunting me; I try not to give it strength by thinking about it but I cannot ignore it. I feel the fight going on inside of me. I only feel vital, well and healthy when I am being physically active, I helped a friend pack and clean for a move. I rearranged at the studio, cleaned, moved things around. You would think with that physical activity along with teaching and walking I could sleep. But it is like if I fall asleep that stalker is going to sneak out. My body and mind are on alert like not letting the guard down. Anything now that happens sticks with me, nothing runs off me, it is like it is on replay; a lab result, a discussion, a decision, a dilemma, nothing will move aside. Tonite I am ruminating, I think about my son Nick, I love that kid, he will be fine without me, but just knowing that he will have that feeling of not having that person who loves you more than anything, who will do whatever it takes and be there for you always. I miss my Mom every day, but I know life goes on, the sun continues to rise even without her. Nick and I have a wonderful special relationship, we are friends, can share ideas and ideals, laugh and not judge, just enjoy each other and what we get from each other. I know he will miss me but I know he will be OK. I wish him love and happiness. I'm happy to know he has someone who loves him. And my wonderful John who I love so much, all he ever wanted was to be loved, to have someone to share his life with. 'We have such a great life together, living in an idealic place, we spend time together, just being. I have to admit the thought of leaving him makes me feel jealous. The thought of him making love to another woman makes me crazy. How shallow I am; he is a vital strong passionate loving man, and an amazing lover, I don't want to share that even in death. But I don't want him to be alone, I want him to find someone to love and have a great life. But yikes, the thought of his being in bed with another woman, OMG, maybe just that idea alone is enough to make me fight like hell and say hell no, I ain't going anywhere. You son of a bitch stalker, stay the hell away.

I met a young woman at the studio on Sunday who is suffering from illness, autoimmune diseases. WE commiserated as in both cases it is our own bodies who are the enemies, we are fighting against ourselves as it is our own body who is the suicide attacker. How messed up is that! That meeting and discussion did prompt me to think how we need a class simply "Yoga to Cope". I really feel yoga helps me cope every day, whether it is something worrisome, or just to stop and take another breath. It is about living and no matter where we are in our journey we need to do that.

Last night John and I had an amazing kayak outing, explored an area we had never been before and as we meandered around had no idea how to back track out and hopefully would empty out eventually into the Gulf. Well it did, and wow. Currents, head wind but amazing. We made it home as the sun was setting, and we felt like adventurers, victorious. Yesterday I felt good all day, wow, although on Wednesday night while coming home from the cancer support group I felt a discomfort in my right arm pit. As I poked around I found a hard knot, in my mind nodes aren't round, and cancerous nodes usually aren't tender, they are usually painless. But PET scan on this coming Wednesday so all will be revealed if something is happening. I had vowed to not check my body, check my weight but the not knowing is the worst part. I got on the scale today and what most women would be thrilled to see I felt a hole in the pit of my stomach. I have lost weight. I am not dieting, I eat pretty much the same thing every day, it is not a calorie dense diet, fruits, veggies, gluten free, some eggs and fish but not daily. I do indulge in coconut milk ice cream at night with a half of a gluten free brownie muffin. So, weight loss is a bad sign. I admit that I feel depressed most of the time and my appetite isn't as great as it has been lifelong. So is it my head, my body, or this suicide bomber. Well, I will find out on 9/25. Today is a new day, as I felt so good yesterday today I feel anxious. Damn, is it my body is it my head.? Yikes, now I really understand how those with depression have so many somatic complaints. But I rolled out my yoga mat on the lanai by the pool; and on the mat, I feel alive, I feel healthy and well, happy and whole. I question how I can be sick while I am so physically strong, stable and focused. Yikes this head trip thing isn't like the head trips I took as a teenager with chemicals. This is a head trip of hell.

My 63rd birthday is coming up on 9/27, and I am going to make it to that regardless of the PET result. If you had asked me end of last year when I got diagnosed, I would have told you I would likely not be around for the event. My wonderful John has made reservations for us in Savannah, GA to spend the weekend. I am so looking forward to it. We have been sleeping separate now for months because of this damned insomnia, so regardless of my sleeping I will be happy to be there beside my man. As there won't be any demands of the studio, work, regular life we can be on our own time doing what we wish, holding hands, laughing, crying, loving. Whatever life points us to. And regardless of the PET results we will be making plans, just that the plans will differ based on the result.

September 17, 2015 Monday sept 21 is world gratitude day. so instead of waiting til Monday I would like to express my gratitude today. Every day is a gift and it was made even more wonderful by having a great phone conversation with my Nick Tumminello this afternoon and then taking a nice walk with my John when he came home from work. A gentle drizzle mist fell with a soft breeze. I am so grateful, I am so fortunate to have 2 great guys to love and be loved by.

September 21, 2015 World Gratitude Day

www.daysoftheyear.com

https://www.daysoftheyear.com/days/world-gratitude-day/
I always felt grateful but it now has an even deeper meaning to me. Now I notice and feel grateful for the little things that I may have overlooked before.

9/22 Tomorrow is the PET scan, I am quite anxious, although in another sense relieved that the result will be known in 2 days and maybe I can be a little less neurotic for a little bit. My wonderful John is going to take me, since I won't be able to eat or drink anything beyond tonight I will be a bit shaky tomorrow both emotionally and nutritionally. Just having my John taking me makes me feel secure and loved. And I am requesting that he gets me a chai to great me when done. I am charging up my MP3 to play Snatam Kaur and getting my eye pillow out to use while in the scanner. They begin by injecting a radioactive glucose solution, then you sit to let it distribute around the body. Once at the scanner, you are strapped down and go into the tube, it is a 20-minute process and quite freaky if you open your eyes. So, with the eye pillow and Snatam Kaur I am assured to turn inward, find my calm and just breathe. The first PET taught me what I needed to do, the second PET went by quickly, and I am sure this one will also. Now the real stress will be waiting to get the results on Friday with Dr. Wenk. And my John is going with me, I need him there, but need him for so much more. I love that man and regardless of the results, we will have a great weekend in Savannah. I especially look forward to sleeping with him, not having any time crunch to go in the morning. I miss him so much that I now sleep separate, I cocoon myself in the spare bedroom, closed door, quiet, dark cool. Without disruption and disturbance, I am getting some sleep with help of magnesium, melatonin and Lorazepam. I never had insomnia except a few nights a year, never had anxiety or felt overwhelmed with stress or worry. But this is the new normal, yikes.

I received a call today from my original oncologist's attorney, asking if I would be willing to come to a hearing in his noncompete case. This is a crazy situation he is who I have thanked for saving my life and being there for me til my last chemo. When I became aware he was changing practices he stated clearly, he would not be able to see me in his new practice and that was that; the only thing I can equate the feeling to is when I was 3 years old and I was taken from my mother's arms to have a tonsillectomy. The sense of insecurity and panic. The thought that a business decision was going to keep me from the man who gave me rebirth. He is such a good man, a really good doc, he doesn't deserve that hassle. The point is care of the patient, and with his noncompete being he cannot care for his patients, it is a direct harm, insult, and slam at those that he has earned their trust, respect and dependence.

September 23, 2015 I'm here to get my scheduled PET scan hard to believe it's been 6 mos. since my last showing I was in remission. I am anxious but more with when I get the results on Fri. Admittedly I've become neurotic over every sensation and since my blood work hasn't been all good I'll at least know. I think it is the not knowing that makes me fear the worst.

September 27, 2015 My John and I have just returned from a 2 night get away in Savannah to celebrate life, still in remission and today is my 63rd birthday. So, a real yahoo because honestly, I wasn't so sure I would be around to turn 63. If you go to Savannah you must try the restaurant Pacci, at the Brice Hotel. The food was awesome, went there for lunch yesterday and brunch this morning before we left to head home. And kudos to John, he drove his Audi, ran beautifully (for those that know John and his Audi adventure, you understand this).

Received my PET scan report on 9/25, still clear, in remission, a big yay. I decided to live life and stop thinking about and writing about this suicide bomber, tormentor called cancer. John and I went to Savannah for a weekend, try to reclaim "us", the insomnia took its toll, couldn't sleep, yikes, so we returned home a day early. a big frustration is the effect on our sex life. We remained active all thru chemo, and now all these months later, there is a problem. What the hell is that about. Can't sleep in the same bed - can't sleep period.......

October 15, 2015 This has definitely been reinforced into me over the last 11 months. And yes 11 months as it was November last year I started the journey into medical consumerism with "the great spleen adventure". If I focus on what was I will not be too happy, if I focus on what may happen I will be a stress cadet, but today is beautiful, the sun is rising, my hair is growing, awoke to my husband by my side, I will be teaching at 10 and surrounded by beautiful spirits and support. Life is a beautiful thing. So grateful for today. Living and Loving IT. The present is truly a GIFT. It is NOW.

I started having some nose bleeding, first noticed on my return flight from MN in June, didn't give it a thought, was dry, I was on blood thinners, etc. And intermittently would have some blood but again, didn't get my attention as I have a life long history of nose/sinus troubles. But over the last week it has become an issue. I am now 3 weeks off Xarelto, yay, and suddenly there is constant blood in my right nostril. A year ago, the thought of cancer in my nose would have never been a thought but now all I can think about is that it is cancer, they are going to cut half my face away, etc. I have an appt with the ENT on Monday 10/19, just get it checked. But now everything looks like cancer to me, the fear of that pervades everything. As for the insomnia I am not needing to take the Ativan which makes me happy as I was tired ALL day from it. But I awaken around 3, fall back to sleep sporadically and then awake for good at 5. But I am falling asleep, taking only Melatonin and Magnesium. I feel so much better with that. Hard to believe when I realize it is 11 months since the adventure began. It was Nov 17 when my spleen ruptured. How things have changed not just from having had surgery, becoming a medical consumer, but now life has such a different flavor. Always having this thing hanging over me. But I am so grateful that I feel good (in the new normal way) I am active and sporting my new short silver do well. My body is firming up again, I am feeling pretty strong and the anxiety isn't nearly as bad. But now with worrying over the nose bleed thing is bringing those other things up again, I feel my inner body jumping around, hard to focus and my GI is running wild. Ugh. Gotta remind myself to just breathe and be in the now. Today is good.

Visit to the ENT yesterday and good news. Although my sensibilities and medical experience told me the nasal blood was a small septal area likely from dryness and mucosal thinning I couldn't help but fear the worst.

October 21, 2015   I love this. Probably wouldn't have last year but I really appreciate it now. My hair is white silver framing my face and salt/pepper elsewhere. It is short and I get compliments on it, that cracks me up. What I've noticed is the light hair around my face is less contrast with wrinkles so my skin looks firmer. And when I look in the mirror now I acknowledge success in making it to be a year older as that was in jeopardy.

October 25, 2015   What an amazing 2 days at this conference. The presenters were those that do and publish the research and are on the forefront of integrative medicine. So grateful I had the opportunity to attend and met some amazing folks. Now it is up to me to put a program together to help those touched by cancer at home. Learned, reaffirmed and feel like I did some personal growth and healing. Amazing what they are doing at MD Anderson with yoga and the research on going. I always enjoy soaking up the info and feel empowered to bring this home to so many who will benefit from it.

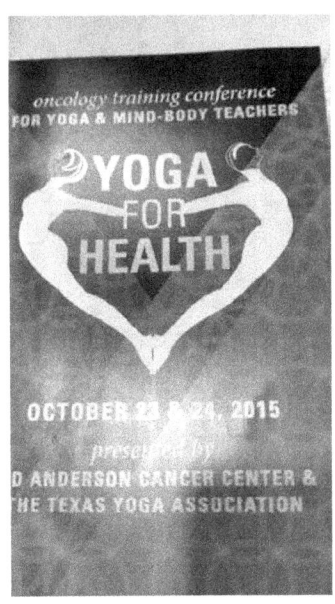

I am here in Houston attending Yoga for Health Integrative Oncology by the MD Anderson Cancer Center. An impressive group of presenters, PhD's and MD's who are doing the research, getting the grants and publishing the papers on the benefits of mind body practices in cancer care. I enjoy getting the info in a scientific fact-based fashion as I believe in yoga, breath work and meditation and its positive effects. And how I know it has helped me in this journey. We did some great meditation and breath work all day, I felt very focused and calm. Went out to dinner with 2 yoga teachers from Texas but came back with an upset stomach. Didn't finish my food although I was really hungry, went between cramps and going to the bathroom and feeling hungry all night so all that meditation and breath work didn't help me with sleep. Had to breakdown and hit the Ativan as I needed to get some sleep.

We are starting the day today with a yoga class perhaps some movement will help.

October 28, 2015 I just returned from an MD Anderson Integrative Medicine workshop on Yoga for Health. And the fact that Yoga is such an important part of my life not just professionally but personally, as a cancer survivor, medical professional and yoga teacher, A trinity of knowledge.

November 5, 2015

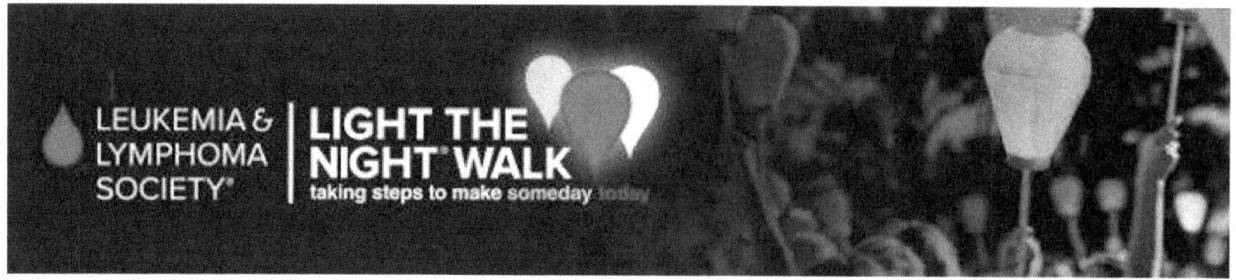

Please visit us at To Each His OM/Flow Yoga vendor booth at Rasa Lila. We are donating a portion of all our proceeds from that day to the Leukemia and Lymphoma Society/Light the Night Walk that evening. This is personal for me. Lymphoma is an equal opportunity blood cancer, of course being a yoga teacher, vegetarian, and living a good life didn't prevent it from happening to me. Please help. Namaste

November 8, 2015   I can't thank everyone enough who contributed to the Leukemia & Lymphoma Society Light the Night walk. The event raised $400k and thank you to Denny, Elaine Davidson-Peebles, Barbara E. Grant, Jack & Carol Tracht-Kader and my John for being there at my side carrying red lanterns signifying they are being there as supporters of someone in the fight. Yellow lanterns were carried by those in memory of someone and I got to carry a white lantern as the survivor. When I was given the survivor shirt, which I wore proudly, and the lantern I got choked up. Sometimes I go thru my day without giving it all a thought. But I had that moment accepting the shirt and lantern with extreme gratitude. That I was truly walking the walk. — feeling thankful.

November 16, 2015   This is the one-year anniversary of "the great spleen adventure" and my journey into medical consumerism. So hard to believe that a year has passed since I was in the hospital, under the knife, getting blood transfusions, in ICU and meeting with an oncologist. How my life changed in just a few hours. Once I received the correct diagnosis (as the original one was incorrect) I questioned whether I would still be here this one year later. Thank you for such great care, love and support I received. And for having learned the tools (yoga) to help me thru each day. I am here today and so grateful for it.

November 17, 2015

Why I'm Quitting (and You Should, Too)

www.wanderlust.com

It took life threatening illness for me to get this. It is so hard for me to explain to my husband why I am good with working medically only one day a week and how I want all the time I need to work on my passions, my programs, and plans. To devote the time to the studio and its needs - this is my time.

November, 26, 2015 This is something that is very pertinent to me right now. It appears my vagal tone is low, I am very aware of it, knowing it is low frustrates and frightens me and that doesn't make it any better for sure. But I am working on helping correct the imbalance and it has made improvement.

Happy Thanksgiving to everyone. And yes, I am really giving thanks. What a ride the last year has been. I've always been aware of my great fortune and been grateful for it. I had 2 wonderful loving and supportive parents, Although I didn't always make them proud and they spent many sleepless nights worrying, I eventually came around to be the person they knew was waiting to blossom. What can I say about my amazing son Nick Tumminello, I ask how did I do that one. My wonderful John, my friends and family, great education, career, live in sunny Florida, Flow Yoga and all the wonderful souls I would have never met had I not taken the Yoga path, my life is easy. So, I reflect that I have had a life of easel this last year was my lesson. Not that I will ever say I am thankful to be given a life-threatening illness, but I am thankful that I've had time to be introspective, to gain a new appreciation, to become more compassionate and understanding. To learn to live a more balanced life. To stop and breath, really embrace the moment, and to look beyond and how I can benefit others' lives. So, for the disease I say, damn you, but for the life experience I say, thank you. And big thanks because I am here living well, loving a lot and working on laughing even more. I don't see my original oncologist anymore (and that's another story) but Dr. Uday Dandamudi thank you. Happy thanksgiving everyone, with gratitude and love Faith

November 27, 2015 Awesome day. Started off with John and I taking an hour-long walk. I then went to the studio to teach our 10 am class. John tried out and signed up for the dragon boat race in the bayou next week. He then went for a bike ride. I met him in Dunedin and we walked the Causeway to Honeymoon Island and back. Now at Frenchy's and they have gluten free beer. Yay. Life is awesome. And I got to speak to my son Nick Tumminello. I am a lucky happy girl.

November 30, 2015 One of the healing gifts I gave myself was having my 2001 Honda Accord repainted. Florida sun burns the paint off of cars and I had it repainted in 2008 which began disappearing 2 years ago. So, one month repainted and first coat of wax. I'm Happy. It only just turned 100k miles and is a 5-speed manual. Not ready to relinquish driving a stick and being car payment free. It's been a great car since coming home to me in June 2001 wanna drive it til the wheels fall off.

A big thanx to Kalamity Kat Rooney, LMT for a great relaxation massage last afternoon. I was truly blissed out and got a great night's sleep. Thank you soooo much. If I could only do that every evening my insomnia would be a no issue *smile emoticon*, I can only wish.

December 10, 2015   got this wonderful quote in an email I received from Anand Mehrotra. I think it is perfect. "If you have never been called crazy in your life, you have never really lived" - Anand Mehrotra

December 24, 2015 It was one year ago today I got the definitive diagnosis and knew 2015 was going to begin unpleasant and the end result questionable; but today I am eager for the new year as I am healthy and looking forward to all good things

December 25, 2015 This year was definitely more upbeat than last year. Last year I referred to our dinner as "the last supper" as it was going to be the last for spicy food and an accepting GI tract as I was about to begin the chemo regime the following day. So, this year lots of hot sauce for me, _smile emoticon_

December 29, 2015 (in response to a post about chemo) that is true but without the chemo most of us would die much quicker. So unfortunately, the reality is die sooner or later and with some luck you get a nice interlude and get some more meaning and joy out of life. For the cancers that are directly related to lifestyle, no excuse for those folks. It pisses me off to see people smoking etc. Unfortunately for those of us who got the bad juju somewhere along the line we gotta just do the best we can. I wouldn't be here today if I didn't do the chemo, but I recognize and accept it may just be an intermission. But life is worth it.

December 30, 2015   and not all cancers are lifestyle related and we have no clue why, so we can't prevent something we don't know the cause. so, prevention of what we can absolutely

This post has bothered me since I first saw it and I must speak. #1 we will continue to see a huge rise in cancer cases, we will see people dying 10-15 years after treatment, we will see toxicity, we will see an increase in treatment related cancers, myelodysplastic syndromes, and other cancers for a few BIG reasons. People first off are living longer in general then they did before and the BIGGEST risk factor for cancer is age as we are exposed to the stressors that cause DNA damage. Yes, DNA damage, Cancer is damaged DNA so chemo and radiation causing DNA damage, duh!!!! Also, people are living longer with chronic illnesses that would have killed them off before. With those chronic illness they are taking medications, by definition a medication (which is chemo therapy) is a poison as it alters a bodily process. so, with that there are likely cancers from everyday drugs, they are chemicals and we know some chemicals are carcinogenic. We are also getting remissions in cancers that we didn't get before, for instance my cancer, Non-Hodgkin's Lymphoma had a 40 % remission rate just 15 years ago but that is now up to 70% so lucky me as I benefited from a monoclonal antibody that is now used in the cocktail. So, people are living longer with the cancer so the other things can exert themselves. I recognize I may die from heart failure as one of the drugs I received is cardio toxic, and yes, if I don't relapse, the suicide bomber doesn't decide it wants to come back for an encore, my bone marrow may fail and I get taken out there, another bone cancer yay. The thought is now living with cancer like other chronic illness because cancer is us, not an invasion from an outside force but our own body going haywire and becoming suicidal. No, it isn't a fungus or a virus and yes maybe those stressors were significant in the process, but there are no other options. to kill the cancer we are killing ourselves, just hopefully the bad guys only. If flax, hemp, green tea, turmeric, alkalinity, meditation etc. cure cancer they would also prevent it and I wouldn't have gotten it. Plenty of charlatans out there, but what we got is what we got. So, from someone with a medical degree, who has become a personal expert on my cancer, integrative options and from a standpoint that I said in the past I would never do chemo, well when it came down to do or die I did and I am alive. Cures for cancer are not here yet, and will likely never be, remissions are where we are and some remissions are brief and some last for life. But for all of us who live with this demon, the truth sucks, I see people all the time who say I don't want to poison my body, and yes, I agree. And you should have a choice, I chose to give it my best shot, chemo it was, I continue with hemp, flax, etc. but I am glad I did because I would not be here writing this today. And I accept that it may be an intermission but it was WELL WORTH it.

<u>December 31, 2015</u> Perfect. And it was that special family that got me thru 2015. Thank you to my "sister" Carol Tracht-Kader who so lovingly cared for me, cooked for me, took me where I needed to go during my adventure into medical consumerism. And Ingrid Wahling whose love for Dock Dog was unwavering even with her own health issues, she was always there for us. And my wonderful friend Kim Weierheiser whose smile and cheer and the surprise Tom Yum soup always perked me up. She kept me going seeing patients, feeling needed vital. So, my family of wonderful friends, thank you so much, I do hope in 2016 I can give you laughter, joy, happiness only. As I plan to be around for a while making all that misery worth it. And to my wonderful husband John, and my amazing son Nick Tumminello you guys are my rock, love you.

Section Two

My Tools of Healing Through Cancer to Living Life to The Fullest

When diagnosed with, being treated for, or living with a life altering and life-threatening illness, there are a number of problems that the patient/survivor and/or caregivers suffer with. These problems can occur individually, sequentially and in combination. Our medical system focuses on the diagnosis, evaluations and treatments of the conditions and judges response to care based on testing, symptoms and progression/remission of the disease process.

Patients and/or caregivers may often overlook many complaints or signs as either a part of the disease, or not important enough to mention, and all too often, they don't want to trouble the medical professionals with these issues. But there are a multitude of concerns that when ignored over time can manifest into poor treatment response and/or a loss of quality of life. Many patients may initially do well and may start noticing changes and concerns once treatment has concluded and remission has been achieved. And we can never discount the stress on family members and caregivers as they bear the burden of the patient's illness plus their responsibilities in care. As a group, caregivers are often overlooked but whose care and diligence are essential and can lead to success or failure. And those on the front line of treatment, infusion nurses, radiation techs, phlebotomists, even the smiling front desk greeters, financial advisers and check out staff, are part of this caregiving team. These caregivers see the patients on a regular basis; spend time with them and many times getting to know them and their families intimately, hearing the real story of what is going on. They, too, need to care for themselves so they can continue to care for others.

Even if we have been given an all clear with the disease, there are other issues that may be ahead of us... And for my journey, I always have this to look forward to: According to a study published in *Cancer*," Patients with diffuse large B cell lymphoma (DLBCL) are at an elevated mortality risk from non-cancer causes even after the disease is cured,. risk of death from factors other than this malignancy, including treatment-related side effects and disease-induced immunosuppression., blood disease ((highest risk), infection, gastrointestinal disease, vascular diseases, and lung disease between 0 and 59 months post-diagnosis were particularly high; after 59 months these risks were lower, though not non-existent." All the more reason to use every tool available for me to stay as healthy as possible and live the best life possible.

"The harder you fall, the heavier your heart; the heavier your heart, the stronger you climb; the stronger you climb, the higher your pedestal." **Criss Jami, Killosophy**

"Proof is boring. Proof is tiresome. Proof is an irrelevance. People would far rather be handed an easy lie than search for a difficult truth, especially if it suits their own purposes."
Joe Abercrombie

The truth is, this journey sucks. I am not giving you a "the truth to healing yourself from cancer.... blah blah blah". That crap is out there. So, buyer beware. I do not believe in any conspiracy theories, I do, though, believe we are not being treated holistically, as there is more than just the drugs and tests. This is about living and living our best life possible whether you are still free of disease, dealing with disease and its wrath or on the road to recovery. Each day is a gift, there are no refunds, credits or exchanges, so we might as well make the best of it.

It is normal for us to look for a quick answer, something for us to grab a hold of and hope it takes us where we want to go. But the reality is this is life, a roller coaster ride of ups and downs, twists and turns, stops and starts, and even being turned upside down and inside out. So, whatever you do, where ever you go for help, use critical thinking skills to disseminate sense from the snake oil sales as there are plenty of charlatans out there.

I am giving you what I found helped me, I did my research, I questioned, I acted. And I hope if you decide to try some of what I offer you will find your best self-possible. I am not selling you a cure, I am only offering some tools that I discovered to help each day be meaningful and worth living. Some is personal inspiration, trial an error, self-discovery and research on the subject matter. Always consult your medical professional, and don't forget to sprinkle everything with laughter, love and gratitude.

"A lie can travel half way around the world while the truth is putting on its shoes."
Charles Spurgeon

"Write down the thoughts of the moment. Those that come unsought for are commonly the most valuable." **Francis Bacon, Sr.**

Journaling

There are so many changes that take place; physical, emotional, spiritual. Some can be at diagnosis, before treatments begin, during treatment, and afterwards, anytime in the journey. Regardless of its chronology it is so difficult to synthesize everything, differentiate between what is a normal expected sensation to a reaction that is out of the ordinary. This is a journey that doesn't come with directions, you are your own guide. And this is a great time to write down your feelings, concerns, fears, experiences, the joys and gratitudes. Maybe wanting to remember a special moment, event or a person, to circumvent memory issues; because once that time is gone those thoughts may be gone too. And it is helpful to read that journal later to reconnect, validate, and maybe get that reassurance of your strength and fortitude. Without that journal I wouldn't have been able to write this book. And each time I read my journal, I thought, yikes, I forgot about that, or OMG.

If you are undergoing treatments, whether drugs, surgery, radiation, you will find the journal helpful in recognizing how long certain symptoms last, when they usually improve or resolve, and any associations that can be drawn. This can help us in planning our day to day activities as well as reassure ourselves and others that this has been an expected and normal feeling. And, again, because there is so much to remember and understand, this can be a valuable tool to share with medical providers when things seem to be out of the ordinary or worse than customary. As a medical practitioner it makes things clearer when they are documented in a concise, clear manner guiding me to appropriate care.

(During my chemotherapy I journaled my emotional and physical state. My emotions, energy level, appetite, weight, swelling, sleep, discomforts and other physical symptoms, which developed a very predictable pattern. I gained 5 pounds the week of chemo as I was on high dose steroids for 5 days, I had insatiable cravings for potatoes, my legs swelled up and were doughy, I couldn't sleep and felt unsteady on my feet. 24 hours after completing the steroids, I started a withdrawal from them feeling weak and urinating nonstop losing the 5 lbs. And once that was over I was functional until the next round. When I didn't feel good on what I called my bounce back day, and I REALLY didn't feel well, I knew something bad was wrong. And I was right; I had a blood clot in my lung and spent 3 days in the hospital. So, it was in that understanding and monitoring, having the awareness and recognizing what was out of the ordinary, that made the difference my getting prompt care. And with that a good outcome.)

I had almost overlooked the journaling to be included in this book, but while writing this book my son's then girlfriend's grandmother was diagnosed with Lymphoma. We had been in contact every few days and she shared with me how she was feeling and her concerns with her blood pressure which up until she began treatment had been well controlled. I suggested journaling the time and reading of the blood pressure and the timing of her blood pressure medication to see any pattern. It tickled my brain how important this can be. (Thank you, Carmela, for letting me be part of your journey, we never met but texted and phoned. Carmela was not as lucky in her battle with the evil Big L.)

"When you write down your ideas you automatically focus your full attention on them. Few if any of us can write one thought and think another at the same time. Thus, a pencil and paper make excellent concentration tools." **Michael Leboeuf**

"He who takes medicine and neglects to diet wastes the skill of his doctors." **Chinese Proverb**

Nutrition

Evidence suggests that simple lifestyle changes can dramatically reduce the risk of cancer. Results of a recently published study that followed 343,150 people for 5 years found a significant reduction in cancer incidence among those who maintained "healthy behaviors: low alcohol intake, non-smoking, healthy BMI [body mass index], physical activity and a healthy diet.

Enough cannot be said about eating a nutritious clean diet. We are so bombarded by fast and packaged foods, foods with artificial ingredients that are unrecognizable by our body, fillers, fats, sugars, and preservatives. Considering that during cancer treatment and a considerable while afterwards, our liver and kidneys are working overtime filtering out the chemicals/drugs-toxins; adding more junk puts even more strain on our already overtaxed organs. And, of course, consuming alcohol is straining our liver even more. Now I never shun away from a good glass of wine or bubbly but we must consider what is happening in our bodies. All drugs are filtered by either our liver or kidneys, chemotherapy (chemicals) so it doesn't have to just be cancer treatment. We are organic beings, and I am not referring to the organic food industry, but our makeup, the makeup of the animals, flora and fauna around us are organic beings. Our body is geared to process nutrients from organic sources (organic in their chemical makeup from natural vs man made sources) so when we introduce those other non-organic ingredients the body has to work to filter it, detoxify it and rid it from the body; sometimes it just stores it because it can't figure out what or how to do anything with it. And this is a theory being considered as a factor contributing to our overwhelming obesity, autoimmune and cancer problems. We also experience a disruption in the function of our digestive system thru changes in our gastric and oral mucosa, the gut flora, and motility. These changes can inhibit the production of digestive enzymes which breakdown our food into usable absorbable nutrients and help regulate the natural Ph (acid balance), breakdown the lining of the gastrointestinal tract which begins at the mouth and ends at the anus(rectum), These changes can cause mucositis which is a painful breakdown of the lining of the mouth making eating painful and difficult or, experiencing the change in how the nutrients are absorbed thru the thinning and breakdown in the stomach and intestines further complicating the situation. And then we may not get the movement of the food and waste as we should (motility). This can result in reflux, constipation, bloating, nausea and even diarrhea, each having its own impact on the body and life in general. Even if we are able to eat without difficulty, getting the nutrition to heal and restore can be a challenge, so limiting the amount of pre-packaged and/or fast foods and drink and those that list chemicalized ingredients may be beneficial. Have you ever looked at the ingredients on a can of liquid protein meal replacement or supplement? It can be Scary!

We must also understand, as well, that just taking supplements to counter this is not always advisable and getting direction from your healthcare provider is a must. Some supplements can counter act the effect of our treatments or at least compete with the medications, and then some can be taken in too high dosages then accumulating in the body leading to toxic levels. But there is increasing evidence there is an association with certain nutrients of their contribution in syndromes, diseases and prognosis. 'There is increasing evidence of nutrition and lack of certain vitamins being associated with inflammation causing a myriad of physical and mental health issues. We do not want to feed disease; we want to feed our body to be strong and to be whole. It was said by the ancient Greek physician *Hippocrates "Let food be they medicine and medicine be thy food."*

More and more people, even in the absence of illness, are becoming aware of how certain foods make them feel, may disagree with them, or may cause them some unpleasant issues. These can be anywhere from bloating, heartburn or reflux, cramping, gas, diarrhea, headaches, weight gain, sleepiness, in my case mouth sores (aphthous ulcers) and joint pain. If you can associate any of these with foods, these are definitely ones to stay away from. But if you do get a craving you may need to nurture that but avoid daily indulgence. Foods often associated with these effects are fast foods (and during chemotherapy and radiation concern for food borne illness needs to be considered), these high fat, low nutrition and chemical laden foods can be harbingers of numerous issues, inflammatory foods are often thought to be red meats, dairy products and for some gluten; theses can cause any number of problems. Some research suggests that meat (animal products) increases a microbe in the gut that causes inflammation. Lactose in milk and dairy products is a large, fermentable carbohydrate and wheat even with those who do not have celiac disease, may be sensitive to gluten-containing foods which have a high fermentation in the gut.

"If you can't pronounce it, don't eat it" *Should be **Common sense*** Do read labels, but remember real food like fresh produce doesn't have labels; an apple and broccoli speak for themselves, as does a piece of fresh fish or a chicken breast. And if you are getting a protein supplement to make the protein shakes I recommend, get the one that is free of the chemical names you can't pronounce. Just pick up a can of some nutritional food replacement drinks and read the labels – I feel it is what we should try to avoid to prevent illness, certainly not the ingredients we want to put in our body when we are already compromised.

A note to this section and subject, I worked on this writing while doing three transatlantic sailings on Royal Caribbean's Navigator of the Seas and Rhapsody of the Seas. Watching people wait for the elevators complaining that they take so long while only needing to go one or 2 floors, the stairs are readily available. While in the Windjammer (cafeteria dinning venue) people are loading their plates with fried foods, heavy starchy foods and sweets. Not unusual to see a plate with pancakes, French toast, a pastry, bacon and sausage, lunch is a repeat just with lunch style foods. Many are obese, unable to move beyond a waddle and most are younger than me and I am sure most are not post chemo. I, on the other hand, load my plate with fresh fruit and it is available at every meal, fresh and cooked veggies; lean proteins such as fish and chicken are always available for meat eaters, a cup of green tea and I do indulge in a small gluten free chocolate sweet when available. And we had a blast on the dance floor after climbing the stairs of those 10 decks. Every morning I go out on deck 5 port side forward to communicate with the wind and water, do a yoga practice, and later in the day walk the length of the ship repeatedly. Go to the gym for weights or use the deck for a body weight work out. I am not just alive – I am truly LIVING)

Our Digestive System is to assimilate the food we eat and convert it into energy. It is our second line of defense against infection, supports our microbiome, interacts with our endocrine, nervous and circulatory systems. Because our ability to digest, absorb and assimilate is compromised during treatment, clean energetic sources of nutrition is paramount.

Do be aware there are many sources out there that tout cancer cures with diets, drinks and supplements. There is no reliable statistics to their efficacy. My recommendations are not aimed at curing but of strengthening, sustaining and rehabilitating ourselves thru nutritive tools. It is well known that eating mostly nuts, bean, legumes, grains, vegetables and fruits with less reliance on animal-based products is a healthy diet, often referred to as the Mediterranean Diet (also considered a more alkaline diet). This is not to be confused with the claims of an alkaline diet, drinking alkaline water, alkalinizing the body to cure cancer. (Cancer cells create an acidic microenvironment due to a high metabolic rate. Cancer cells can't live in a highly alkaline environment, but neither can healthy cells. Your body works to keep pH levels constant, and changing your diet is not going to substantially change the pH levels of your blood, which are tightly regulated by the kidneys and lungs regardless of foods consumed. The pH of bodily fluids, such as saliva and urine, does change temporarily depending on the foods you eat, but that doesn't affect blood pH levels (or, hence, the environment of cancer cells in the body). In fact, any significant deviation in blood pH levels can cause serious, even life-threatening conditions known as acidosis (low pH) or alkalosis (high pH) So buyer beware!

There has been an increased understanding of the microbiota (gut flora) and its importance not just for digestion but for total health and wellness. Research now suggests that the microbiota which includes bacteria, fungi, and viruses, plays an important role in carcinogenesis, cancer progression, and treatment response. Most of the evidence for the association between the microbiota and cancer comes from animal studies, some human studies have supported these findings. The microorganisms present within the human body is 100 times greater than human genes. Because the microbiota is instrumental in multiple normal human processes, the permanent deviation of the composition and function of the microbiota and their relationship to its host, is associated with multiple pathologies. One being cancer. Some studies have demonstrated that response to chemotherapy may be modulated by the gut microbiota.

"Understanding is a three-edged sword: your side, their side, and the truth."   **J. Michael Straczynski**

Food not just feeds the body but fuels the mind, to help maintain a mental environment conducive to healing and living our best life possible. **Unknown**

The Goal of Nutrition is:

*To sustain the body during treatment
 *Provide a base to help restore and recuperate after treatment
*To provide the cellular energy to regenerate what has been lost both from the disease and the treatment
*To prevent, minimize or better tolerate side effects of treatment

Foods:

If you are undergoing chemotherapy or radiation, are on immune suppressants or have a poor immune system, you must employ great caution with food hygiene. Caution with the ice from restaurants, motels etc. as these are made in big machines that are known to harbor bacteria. My best friend is a microbiologist and the stories of contamination she can share, it is amazing any of us survive. Fruits and vegetables (even those that are bagged and state prewashed) can harbor bacteria, as appears in the news time to time with bagged lettuce and spinach. Only you can assure cleanliness. And be cautious about the surfaces your food touches, to assure they are clean and sanitized. The same can be for probiotic supplements or foods with probiotics in them; in a healthy individual these are beneficial bacteria to promote a healthier digestive system but can overwhelm an immune compromised individual. On a normal basis, a healthy person will not get sick from this common type of contamination but when our immune system is compromised these small invaders can mean life and death.

(When I was getting chemo, I became fanatical about kitchen cleanliness. Made my husband crazy as this was from a person who shunned hand sanitizer saying we need those bugs to keep us healthy. I wouldn't eat the watermelon he cut if he didn't wash the rind completely before cutting it, same with bananas with the peel. It became a neurosis with me but I got thru it without any problem. When we did go out to eat, and there was only one place I would go, a local Thai restaurant that would take caution with my meal, I would roll up the placemat so that the menu didn't touch any eating surface or utensils. I ordered the same thing every time and after a few times they knew not to put anything raw on the plate, ice or lemon in my water. If I touched a menu I would immediately use hand sanitizer. It was a crazy time but the extra efforts were worth it as I avoided any illness, even avoided catching a cold when it was all around me. I am now back to inviting some germs into my body to keep me healthy.)

" Life expectancy would grow by leaps and bounds if green vegetables smelled as good as bacon." **Doug Larson**

Fruits & Vegetables:

Unless you are on Warfarin/Coumadin lots of leafy greens like spinach, kale, brussels sprouts, cruciferous like broccoli and cauliflower, and root veggies like carrots and beets should be eaten daily. Wash all your veggies thoroughly with either a commercially available fruit and veggie wash or make your own. You can use some peroxide and water or a vinegar and water mixture to scrub your veggies. The vinegar and water mixture as a soak works well to remove some of the insecticides/pesticides as well.

Instead of eating these raw, to assure they are free of contamination a brief sterilization in a microwave or steamed on the stove, just enough for the heat to change the texture and get steamy but not enough to destroy all the nutrients. (I think it is called blanching – I barely knew how to turn the stove on before this.) With fruit you make compote, actually very tasty as it brings out the sweetness. (My mother would make a fruit compote on holidays, I don't remember ever eating it, I didn't like how it looked, but that is where I got the idea. It turned out to taste really good and I would put the berry compote on an unsweetened coconut milk ice cream for a treat. Even when being careful with what you are eating, you need a little decadence time to time.) Fruits and veggies that have a skin like melons, kiwi, avocado, and banana do not have to be sterilized as the fruit inside is already clean, it is the skin that is potentially contaminated, so before you cut into it wash it thoroughly first. (My husband John finally got it after my repeated hissy fits.) I still wash my fruit and the skins before cutting into them, just smart, you never know.

Citrus fruits and tomatoes (even tomato sauce) can aggravate the delicate lining of the mouth and stomach causing burning and reflux, so be cautious. Avoid fresh salsa at a restaurant *(I missed that so much)* as it is raw and may not have been cleaned sufficiently before preparation. If the salsa is a commercially jarred product it is generally considered acceptable because everything is pasteurized but may still be an aggravant of the GI track. (I had a passion for tomato sauce during chemo, something about how the taste buds get messed up and I developed reflux, had no discomfort, just lost my voice Went to the ENT, scoped me and said reflux was inflaming my vocal cords. Just add another one to the list. No tomato sauce.)

Nuts are a great source of protein but caution in eating raw nuts, opt for roasted varieties, nut butters or nut milks instead. Using the raw nuts in recipes that are being cooked sufficiently should be OK. (I had always just eaten peanut butter but got introduced to almond butter, really good stuff. And then there is Justin's Chocolate Hazelnut Butter – My Favorite. Thank you Clydean Hoffman, she gave me a jar for Christmas 2013 and it was a wow and remains so now.) Nut intake has been shown to be associated with a reduced risk of type 2 diabetes and insulin resistance as well. And because they now feel that the same factors that cause diabetes and heart disease are the same factors that cause many cancers, lower diabetes risk is a good thing. FYI, peanuts aren't nuts at all, they are legumes.

Eggs can be a good source of protein but should be washed really well before the shell is cracked. Be sure to cook the eggs completely, however you're eating them. No raw eggs while immune challenged. Local free-range chicken eggs are really worth the effort and price, and the chickens are happier too. They are fresh and you can really taste the difference and because the chickens are eating and moving around naturally I suspect they are a bit more nutritious. Do look for hormone and antibiotic free, and if organic free of the pesticides in their feed.

Fish – Try to eat wild caught and avoid those with high levels of Mercury like Tuna and Swordfish. Try to avoid farmed fish which are fed meal, artificial colorants and are swimming in their own feces; antibiotics and chemicals may be added to their water because it isn't their natural environment. And NO SUSHI, no raw during treatment or with any immune compromise. Epidemiologic evidence has shown that fish consumption may have a protective benefit against gastrointestinal cancers, thyroid cancer, multiple myeloma, and childhood leukemia.

Caution with local and raw honey even though it is good in terms of nutrition– commercially available honey usually has been sterilized unless it says raw which is a no no. There is a honey from New Zealand called Manuka Honey, that is actually healing. It is used on wounds and can be very good for GI discomfort. You can get a medical grade, I got it on line and was well worth it for me. I started every morning off with cup of hot water, a spoonful of Manuka Honey and Organic Lemon Juice.

"Let food be thy medicine and medicine be thy food." – Hippocrates

"An apple a day keeps the doctor away" ~Proverb

Some ideas you can add to your day that will soothe you, energize you, and help you heal.

Make your own smoothie in a blender.

Mix a protein powder, flavor of your choosing and watch the ingredients, you want to avoid herbs like ginseng and probiotics if you are on chemotherapy for cancer. They are usually a whey protein, rice, hemp and other plant-based protein, like pea protein. I avoided whey as it is a milk product and I limited my milk during treatment because of the potential to be inflammatory. Add in milks, almond, rice or coconut milk (soy is good as long as there is no problem with the soy estrogen as with a hormone-based cancer or condition). Use a nut butter if you can, I prefer almond butter, it gives flavor and texture (this adds more protein to help rebuild what is being lost in the treatment). Add in fruit and veggies (although you must acquire a taste for veggies in smoothies there are some green powders that work well) that has been steamed/blanched (compote), and or banana, melons (whatever you have). You can also add in some juices, do make sure it is 100% juice and not a juice drink as they usually have a good bit of added sugar.

To add some more nutrition to the smoothie use some beet and carrot juice (use these together unless you like the taste of beets, the carrot juice cuts the beet flavor and can add a little sweetness, you can also add cherry, grape, apple or any berry juice (no more than an ounce of each as juices are higher in sugar). And blend away. A little ice cream (again I prefer coconut milk ice cream) can cool it down, thicken it up and feel like a milk shake instead of a smoothie. You can add ice as long as it is coming from a known clean place.

Watermelon is good for the water content, berries are high in antioxidants (do watch berries, though, as they are high in insecticides, so if you are only going to do one thing USDA organic make it berries and grapes), dark cherries have magnesium which can help with sleep, muscle pain and constipation, bananas have potassium and don't forget the Vit C found in fruits. Add as much or as little of these as you like to taste and texture. Protein powders usually come in chocolate, vanilla and a few in berry. With a little trial and ingenuity, you will discover what flavors go best with what. And you can have variety.

"Sometimes the questions are complicated, and the answers are simple." **Dr. Seuss**

Fruit Compote

This is simple and tasty. If you like apple or cherry pie this is a winner as what you are eating of the fruit in a pie is cooked so this is what a compote is-cooked fruit.

Good combos – strawberries and blueberries; apples with cranberries and rhubarb; apples and pears; or any fruit on its own including apricots, peaches etc. If you can't find the fruits fresh, look for them frozen. Make your compote up small batches at a time as it gets runny and mushy when refrigerated.

Place the fruit for steaming in a glass or stone wear bowl (Do Not use any plastic or Styrofoam) in the microwave and put on high for 20 seconds, check the fruit and see if any pieces have started to lose its shape and consistency, stir and return up to another 20 seconds, repeat as needed. It is done once some pieces soften, careful to not overdo it. You may find more juice in the bowl and it is steaming but it doesn't need to be soupy. I know there is controversy about microwaves, some theories are they are not good and some others have shown that when used properly the nutrients are actually preserved more than conventional cooking. You be the judge. I've not found convincing evidence yet on either side.

On the stove top, place the fruit in a sauce pan on medium heat, keep stirring/tossing the fruit in the pan until softening and steaming takes place. Be careful as this can burn quickly and the sugars from the fruit caramelize. And I hate scrubbing pots, guess that is another reason I prefer the microwave.

Enjoy as a desert alone, in the smoothie, or to accompany a plain yogurt, an ice cream, with a cereal, whatever your imagination leads you to.

Sorry Mom, I never ate your compote, was a kid thing, I thought it looked yuck. But I know you would be happy and proud to know you were the inspiration for my fruit during the chemo. And even happier to know I found it to have and soothing qualities.

Steamed Veggies

Almost any vegetable can be steamed but the key is to steam it and not overcook it. Use the veggies as a meal in itself or as a complement to other foods, and experiment putting veggies into your smoothie. Of course, baking potatoes and root vegetables like beets and carrots is delicious. Garlic, onions, ginger and turmeric are considered in some cultures as healing. Making your plate as colorful as possible to get an array of nutrients. When eating potatoes choose sweet, red and purple over the white as they have more nutrients. Sorry, but white potatoes have all their nutrition in the skin, otherwise not much else in nutrition.

Soups

Start with a broth (your choice, vegetable, chicken or beef) and just put everything in a pot and let it all cook together. The beauty of soups is it is easy and none of the nutrition is lost as it is all cooked into the soup. You can add whatever protein you like, tofu, or a meat of choice as well. Be cautious of using an egg drop that the egg cooks completely. What also makes soup great is you can make a larger quantity and store it in the frig and quickly reheat it for a nutritious snack or meal. I kept soups at the ready all the time. If you are eating store bought soup just read the labels. There are some good organic soups out there and I developed a passion for butternut squash soup that way. Look for those in a container that has a spout that you can close and reuse making it really convenient. Soups really because a go to for me.

Comfort Food

I also found mashed potatoes to be very comforting, we made them in quantity so there was always availability that could be heated up (sweet potatoes mashed was especially good during chemo as it was warm, soothing, sweet and nutritious. And I love hummus, this is so simple with just chickpeas, tahini, lemon, and a little oil, season to taste and use the blender. Can give a little zing but without the burning in the mouth. Foods that have a warm, smooth texture and flavor can be very comforting. (In ancient Indian science, Ayurveda (life science) it is considered calming the out of balance vatta with kapha foods. Vatta is dry and irritated, just what chemo does to you, and kapha is heavy and watery) Comfort foods make us feel safe and at home within ourselves and surroundings. So, treat yourself to feel nurtured both body and mind with comfort foods, you deserve it and need it.

A mention about sugar, try to avoid adding sugar and by all means avoid artificial sweeteners. Honey in its raw state, where it has the most nutrition, can also contain bacteria that can cause problems when immune compromised. If you prefer the taste of honey it needs to be pasteurized but do be aware that that will minimize the nutritional benefit. Stevia is an option as it is a natural/not artificial sweetener but make sure it is just Stevia with no other artificial additives to it.

Why limit sugar? You may have read that sugar feeds cancer, and some recent studies have shown that a certain lung cancer is highly sensitive to sugar. Otto Warburg discovered in the 1920s that tumors take up huge amounts of glucose, which they ferment into lactate rather than respire, The Warburg Effect. Sugar has long been linked to cancer indirectly through associations between obesity and cancer. <u>A 2014 policy paper by the American Society of Clinical Oncology (ASCO) noted that "obesity is a major under-recognized contributor to the nation's cancer toll and is quickly overtaking tobacco as the leading preventable cause of cancer."</u> There is clear correlation between diabetes and cancer, which may be from high blood sugar levels; a direct connection between sugar and tumor growth remains elusive. Some recent clinical trials indicate that "sugar-poor diets are beneficial for recovery of patients with cancer who undergo chemotherapy." Research is looking to understand the primary cause of the high sugar influx into cancer cells not present in regular mammalian cells. Results might offer a new target for cancer treatment.

If you have gotten a PET scan you may understand. During a PET scan you are injected with a sugar solution that carries the radioactive dye. Because cancerous tumors are very metabolically active they take up the sugar solution and that is what is seen on the PET. So, because of this, any sugar ingested will go first to the cancerous cells/tumors because of its metabolism. But cancer will take what it needs to grow anyway, you just don't want to send food directly to it and encourage its growth with the sugar. Also, sugary foods are calorie dense and nutrition deficient so eat foods that will fuel the body's healing and repair instead of empty calories. Ingesting sugar increases insulin secretion and the connection between cancer and insulin is growing but is not yet conclusive. Recent studies have shown that hyperinsulinemia has been shown to have a direct tumor-promoting effect. Hyperinsulinemia also increases insulin-like growth factor (IGF) which is correlated with an increased risk of breast cancer. Moderation is key here as eating a balanced diet with protein, fat, and fiber is recommended so that the sugar is processed more slowly without overproducing insulin.

Meats and dairy, these are thought to be potentially inflammatory which can aggravate pain, they are also acidic so the body will have to work a bit harder to alkalinize and return to the normal pH. A diet consisting of predominantly fruits and vegetables is more alkaline. If you are wrestling with anxiety there is suggestion that meats may aggravate it, as meats help the body produce norepinephrine which is stimulating. As for fats, avocado is an excellent source of fat packed with lots of nutrition; nuts are also a great nutritious source of oil.

Drink lots of water; please avoid sodas, if drinking ginger ale because of nausea watch the quantity because of the sugar content. This doesn't include seltzer water, it is colas. Sodas usually contain lots of artificial ingredients, sugar or artificial sweetener. You can purchase a plain carbonated water and add ginger juice, or any other fruit flavor you wish but use the 100% pure fruit juice to make your own soda water. Be cautious drinking fruit juice itself as it is high in sugar and calories, so just a splash, about an ounce in your smoothie or added to soda water. (Do read the label for sugar content it may surprise you). Limit coffee to one morning cup (again it is very acidic, hard on the body and is known to leach out calcium from the bone-not a good thing when a lot of the drugs do the same) and the caffeine can aggravate anxiety. Opt for a good quality green tea to drink hot or cold. Some studies have shown green tea to lower LDH. Black or other favored teas are good as well, just be aware of the caffeine and its affects.

Nutritional Supplements

Not enough research has been done to really determine the adequate and appropriate use of supplements in healthy populations, as you will notice ranges instead of definitive dosing. There is still so much controversy between the medical and integrative/complementary (formerly referred to as alternative) communities that there is much less known about needs in those compromised by illness and its treatment. There are a few suspected and known concerns with interactions, toxicities and deficiencies but the information is not known or shared universally. There is no consensus about nutritional supplementation and a wide diversity of opinions abound. It is suggested that taking antioxidants will protect the cancer cells so what sounds reasonable may not be so when it comes to cancer. Another word of caution is there is no standardization resulting in lax oversight on the supplement industry so studies have found not just varying amounts in the supplements but sometimes other ingredients completely. So, discussing this with your healthcare provider is paramount so you both can come to a meeting of the minds to best serve your needs.

What is generally considered safe to take but please consult your medical provider first. These are not cures but are being studied and evaluated for their health benefits

Food and Spices as Supplementation

Turmeric

An Indian spice derived from the plant *Curcuma longa*, its active ingredient curcumin, have been studied in a wide variety of diseases, including cancer. In patients with prostate cancer, a small study showed that a supplement of blended pomegranate, green tea, broccoli, and turmeric had a short-term effect on the percentage rise in prostate-specific antigen (PSA). More recently, a study found that a small dose of curcumin significantly decreased the proliferation of glioblastoma multiforme. Another small study showed that oral curcumin reduced the severity of radiation dermatitis in patients with breast cancer.

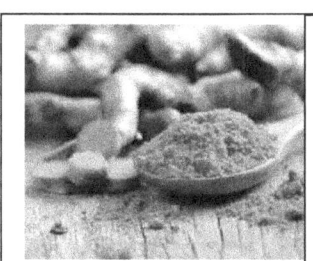

A special thank you to Austin Mascarenhas from Mumbai, Head Waiter on the RCCL Rhapsody of the Seas making sure I have Turmeric at every meal & helping explain to others about its use & benefits

*Caution using Turmeric while on chemotherapy-Supplementation with turmeric and curcumin may not be without harm. Laboratory findings show that dietary turmeric may actually inhibit the anti-tumor activity of chemotherapeutic agents such as cyclophosphamide and doxorubicin. (Unfortunately, while on a cancer fighting regimen you want it to be as active and toxic to the cells as possible to get the bad guys.)

Hemp

Hemp is a very nutritious nut, with a mild flavor and often referred to as hemp hearts. Hemp seeds contain over 30% fat. They are rich in 2 essential fatty acids, Omega 6 and Omega 3. The imbalance of Omega 6 fatty acids in relationship to the lower levels of Omega 3 found in today's Western diets is thought to be one of the primary forces of low-grade chronic inflammation. They are a great source of protein, also a great source of vitamin E and minerals such as phosphorus potassium, sodium, magnesium, sulfur, calcium, iron and zinc. They can be eaten raw, cooked or roasted. Also available in oil form, not used in cooking in the heating process but can be added to foods as a dressing. (I use drizzled on veggies, potatoes, eggs, anything that people would put butter on.) Some studies have noted a decrease in the serum inflammatory marker CRP as well as decreased heart disease and blood clot risk.

Hemp as well as Cannabis is where they extract CBD Oil, that is beyond our writing. As a note Hemp CBD is available over the counter but do be aware there are many growing and extraction methods that are concerning so if you are trying this there is ample information on the Web to educate yourself about what to look for in a CBD Oil

Moringa Olfeira

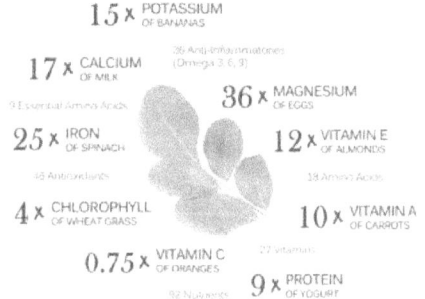

It can be used as a tea, mixed into smoothies or eaten fresh like any other green. And can be grown in warm climates as we grow it in Florida. The powder is readily available as well as tea bags; a few companies are now making products incorporating the Moringa into them. I am so grateful to my next-door neighbor, Lyn, who shares her bounty of Moringa with me, I only need to go next door, cut branches and I have all the Moringa I can use to eat fresh, dry for teas and/or grind to add to smoothies.

Kombucha

Kombucha is a naturally fermented drink with a living colony of bacteria and yeast, a probiotic drink that aids in digestion and gut health. It is fermented, high in acid, contains sugar, vinegar, B vitamins, antioxidants (from the tea) trace amounts of alcohol (a natural product of the fermentation) and some other compounds.

There is a potential danger of home-brewed and unpasteurized kombucha prepared in non-sterile conditions and the risk for unhealthy bacteria getting into the tea. This should be avoided during chemotherapy and if immune compromised.

A safer bet is to go for one that is commercially prepared and pasteurized," says Janet Helm, MS, RD, a Chicago nutritionist and author of Nutrition Unplugged blog. Kombucha contains phytochemicals or phytonutrients that have antimicrobial and antioxidant properties is rich in B-vitamins and folic acid, which is key for helping the body produce and maintain new cells. A big thanks to my neighbor, Kari de Laaf, who loves to share her Kombucha bounty with me so I always have fresh home brewed. And I always keep a stock of my favorite GTS Multi-Green in the frig. I have a patient whose name I cannot use because of HIPPA, who works at a local grocery store and always calls the office to make sure I know it is on sale. So, thank you for that, I really appreciate it.

> "Kombucha is not a cure-all or magical elixir but it does have some beneficial bugs similar to yogurt, kefir, or other probiotic drinks, caution if your immune system is compromised because of the probiotics bacteria".

Gluten-Is it helping you or hurting you?

Whether you're in remission or you've recently been diagnosed with cancer, maintaining a healthy diet is critical to your recovery and well-being. For some aggressive cancers the treatment is equally as aggressive and alleviating symptoms from such treatments is paramount to help a patient feel well. Vegetarian, vegan and low-carbohydrate diets, diets eliminating or minimizing inflammatory foods have long been very popular ways to do this. However, studies are now showing that a gluten-free diet may also help in the fight against cancer.

Gluten is a protein found in wheat, barley, rye and spelt. It is also frequently a source of allergen cross-contamination in many foods. Current statistics show that only five to ten percent of Americans suffer from some form of intolerance to gluten. In spite of those numbers, though, many researchers believe that the vast majority of Americans have trouble with gluten, whether or not they have any obvious symptoms. Again, one of those disputed issues. But I am seeing more and more medical information involving this subject, so the jury is still out.

Even for people with uncompromised immune systems, gluten has been found to have many negative effects on health, digestion and nutrient absorption. Inside the digestive system, gluten forms a thick, paste-like substance that smothers the lining of the intestines. It is believed that this can significantly hinder the availability of nutrients from food. This one fact alone makes a strong case for avoiding gluten during and after cancer. Adequate nutrition is considered an essential part of cancer therapy and recovery.

In individuals with sensitivity to gluten, it can cause serious immune dysfunction. The body interprets the protein as an invader or foreign substance and reacts accordingly. When this happens, the immune system unwittingly attacks the body because there is no real pathogen to fight off. Theoretically, this can increase cancer susceptibility. (With Non-Hodgkin's Lymphoma one of the risk factors is autoimmune disease) When the immune system is occupied with one task, the body is left vulnerable to other illnesses.

For every recognized case of celiac disease, 8 more remain undiagnosed. The reason for this disparity is contingent on the varying presentations of the disease. What was once considered solely a GI disorder, uniformly presenting with diarrhea and malabsorption, has evolved into a multisystem autoimmune disorder with myriad symptoms and signs. In addition, celiac disease is no longer a disorder limited to childhood and adolescence; it has even been diagnosed for the first time in elderly patients. "Atypical" celiac disease—which presents with few or even no GI symptoms or signs—is largely responsible for the increased prevalence of celiac disease today, a great "masquerader," iron deficiency anemia, thyroid disorders, elevated liver enzymes, adrenal dysfunction.   A 5-fold increased risk of non-Hodgkin lymphoma.

(A few years prior to my lymphoma diagnosis my dentist asked me if I had gone gluten free. With a lifelong problem of mouth sores (aphthous ulcers), I had avoided citrus and tomatoes, taken high doses of vitamin C, certain amino acids, antioxidants, used tooth paste without fluoride and sodium laureth, gotten an electric tooth brush to lessen tooth brush "trauma", used different mouth washes, taken antibiotics and anti-virals and all to no avail. Considering I ate a green diet void of meats, minimal dairy and fats only from nuts, seeds and plant sources, I never considered gluten. And I really did enjoy a good loaf of fresh bread especially dipped in olive oil and herbs. Mouth sores wasn't what I had heard as a gluten symptom. But I was open to give it a go, I'd done everything else. So, I tried it beginning that day and from that day forward I never had a mouth sore until I said "hell with it" I want real bread. Well I got a mouth full of sores that lasted a full month of misery. Since that fateful day I haven't had gluten and I've remained sore free even during chemo in which my oral mucosa remained intact. And a risk factor for lymphoma is autoimmune disease, the body is inflamed and always fighting an invader, so maybe all along that was it. More interesting is it was about 4 months later I had the great spleen adventure and my marriage to Big L took place. Being separated from gluten as much as I can, I hope I can keep the inflammatory issue at bay and Big L and I have a lifelong separation. I'd like to say our divorce is final but with cancer you can never say never. Statistics are on my side but not guaranteed.)

Vitamins

Vitamin D – It is hard to sufficiently get enough of it as our body makes it when we are in sunlight. And we know that sun screens limit D absorption. I read something once that said you would have to be outside naked around noon for 2 hours at a location near the equator to absorb enough D. Good excuse to move to your own tropical island :-) It is fat soluble so it is stored in extra body fat and not available for the body to use. Vitamin D's role is to facilitate calcium absorption to fortify our bones; it also is significant in controlling inflammation in the body. The foods we can get it from are Cod Liver Oil, Sardines, Wild Caught Salmon, Mackerel, Tuna, Raw Milk, Caviar, Eggs, Mushrooms and anything that is fortified with Vit D. Epidemiological research suggests that cancer mortality might be higher in northern latitudes where people tend to experience less sun exposure, and hence, lower levels of vitamin-production in the skin. Suggestion of possible biological mechanisms for a relationship between vitamin D and tumor growth, cancer cell inhibition, and anti-inflammatory effects. There is emerging evidence that vitamin D levels in the bloodstream might correlate with lower risks and improved survival in certain cancers, it is not yet clear that dietary supplementation is an effective chemo preventive or cancer-treatment intervention.

B Vitamins help us in cellular metabolism so our body can make energy and repair itself. Deficiencies can result in problems of the nervous system, weakness, tingling/numbness, skin and oral sores, sleep problems, anxiety, depression and anemias. Their food sources are legumes/beans, whole grains, potatoes, and bananas. Because neuropathies are a common side effect and complication of treatments and disease processes, B supplementation may help lessen it a bit as the neuropathy may be worsened by some of the B deficiencies.

Minerals – Be cautious as some minerals can counteract medications by binding them and transporting them out of the body-chelation.

Calcium is an essential nutrient not just for bone and teeth strength but also for the transmission of nerve impulses and muscle contraction (both skeletal muscle as well as cardiac-heart muscle). Many medications disrupt the absorption and utilization of this nutrient. Although the dairy industry wants to encourage you to drink milk for calcium, countries with the highest milk drinking also have the highest rates of osteoporosis so its absorption is what counts. If you are taking certain medications, especially those that affect stomach acid (like a proton pump inhibitor), absorption may be compromised. Calcium absorption is enhanced with Vitamin D and Magnesium.

Magnesium in balance helps work with calcium. Low levels are associated with diabetes, muscle cramping and fatigue. Because its dietary absorption is dependent upon a healthy GI tract, supplementation may be helpful. It is frequently found as a supplement in combination with calcium. Magnesium is also available in a gel that can be used as a muscle/body massage, worked into the feet can help for pain and tingling as well into any muscle tightness and pain. Epson salts is magnesium, so a warm bath/soak can have amazing results. Magnesium also works with motility in the gut so it will help decrease problems of constipation. (If you have ever taken Mag Citrate or Milk of Magnesia, you know what I'm talking about.)

Digestive Enzymes are generally considered safe. As we age most of us lose some of the function involving our natural enzymes that break down the foods we eat. These enzymes breakdown proteins, carbohydrates, fats and dairy. Many people who have reflux may be suffering from low digestive enzymes so the foods eaten are sitting around not being broken down; and there is increased stomach acid being produced to process it. We are usually given acid reducers in one form or another but this can have its own problems (mentioned previously affects nutrient absorption). So, enzymes taken before, with and/or after meals may lessen the problem and the need for an acid reducer.

Herbs can be very powerful so are generally, when used, are done so with great caution. During my chemotherapy treatment I steered away from them because depending upon their timing with chemo can negate some of the chemo effects. (If you are getting chemotherapy for a cancer you want it to be as strong as possible to eradicate the cancer cells). Consult your medical provider about herbs and watch the ingredients of many powder supplements like protein powders as they may have different herbs.

Probiotics are necessary for our gut and total body health. But do be cautious about taking Probiotics as a compromised immune system can get overwhelmed and sick from them, so consult your medical provider. Frequently they will be recommended for diarrhea but usually for only a short period of time. As a general rule, the probiotics in yogurt is minimal and only a few strains; in fact, most of the yogurts are free of many live active cultures. And during the process of digestion, because of the stomach acid breaking down the yogurt, the bacteria is deactivated anyway. (So, the probiotic activity in yogurt is minimal but some can experience a benefit even from that small activity). Kefir, Kimchi and Kombucha are other good natural food sources of probiotics because of their fermentation.

"

From the bitterness of disease man learns the sweetness of health." **Catalan Proverb**

"The part can never be well unless the whole is well." **Plato**

The Practice of Breath, Movement & Mindfulness

The Goal of The Practice Is:
To improve the quality of life
To improve an overall sense of self & well-being
To maintain or gain energy
To encourage healthy activities
To improve mood, calm anxiety/stress
To improve rest/sleep
To improve breathing & ventilation
To improve circulation and assist with lymphatic drainage
To maintain or gain strength and/or mobility
To maintain and gain balance in both body and mind
To maintain and improve focus, concentration and memory
To reduce treatment side effects
*Loss of sensation and discomforts from neuropathy, fatigue, balance challenges, loss of strength and mobility, GI upset, swelling, and a loss of hope and self-esteem. *

The Breath

"Breath is the King of the Mind." **B.K.S. Iyengar**

Everything begins with the breath. When we are fearful and under stress our shoulders tighten, they rise up, our head tilts forward a bit and our chest starts to narrow. This process tightens the chest and decreases the space to breathe into and can cause us to use our shoulders to breath in more air. (using accessory muscles, scalenes) Effective, effortless, full breathing is using the full lung with the breath going into the lung bases first and then filling upwards. So, with shallow breathing we are breathing into the upper lungs rather than the bases and our breath is quick. This can make us feel short of or out of breath discouraging us from moving/exercising even just walking and it can also give us a feeling of tension, pain and anxiety.

There are different approaches to breath work, some to draw more focus, some to cool or heat the body, some to calm the mind and find clarity, some to energize and some to find relaxation. So as each of us is on our own journey, we may find how one breath helps you and not someone else. So, experiment with them, take time, as with any new skill it comes with practice. You may even notice some interesting sensations with your body or mind after doing it the first time, but it will take regular practice for the effects to be lasting. It isn't a quick fix. Once you practice these techniques in a safe quiet space, they will become so natural that when in need you will quickly revert to them to help find natural relief in an unpleasant or unwanted situation. Breath work works quickly, faster than any medication.

Unless specified all the breath techniques are done through the nose. There are a few main reasons for this: first is nasal hairs help to filter the air, second is the nose warms the breath, the third is there is a communication between the nostrils and the brain, where the right side of the brain effects the left side of the body (this includes the nose) and vice versa. The body has a natural cycle of switching which nostril is dominant, this helps keep the nervous system balanced. It is called "nasal laterality". (Good Jeopardy question/answer)

*3 Part Breath – This is good for anyone and can be used anywhere, anytime and in any body position. If you are lying down make sure the body is comfortable, raise your head to a comfortable position, maybe soften and support the knees or

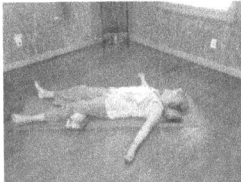

bend the knees with the feet flat on the floor/bed etc. If you are sitting be as upright as possible, with feet comfortably on the floor if in a chair. (Avoid crossing the legs at the knee. If on the floor elevate the buttocks and hips with a pillow and sit with lower legs crossed (easy seated pose) – you can do the same while in a chair which opens the hips. If standing feet should be hip distance apart, toes pointing forward with feet and legs engaged, muscles firm. Stand tall head balancing over the shoulders and shoulders in line over the hips.

Once you find the best position for yourself either close your eyes or keep them soft and focused on one spot. Just take a few natural breaths in and out through the nose, notice any area of tightness or restriction, and notice if the breath is smooth and long, or short and forced, and become aware if the breath is moving low or high into the lungs. Don't change anything just become aware and notice any other sensations or movements that seem to come with it. Notice if your mind is arguing with you or do you have any discomforts. Don't fight with it but acknowledge it and see if you can get more comfortable, making little adjustments at a time.

*Belly Breath - After a few comfortable normal breaths in and out, let your exhalations be long and slow, even making a long slow releasing sigh from your mouth letting go of as much air as possible. With your next in breath (inhalation) through the nose, let the breath go as deeply into the belly as possible, relax your abdominal muscles, even feel your belly expand out a bit and expand rising upwards. Once you fill this space notice if your body is fast to let it go or you can have a second or two pause before exhaling. Then let the breath out slowly and fully through the nose feeling the belly pull back in without making any body tightness or movement into the back. Not forcing the breath in or out, just let it flow in and out. You can place one or both of your hands on your belly to connect to this rise and fall of the breath if this is comfortable for you. Stay here as long as you wish, take your time and enjoy how relaxed you will begin to feel, and you can repeat it as many times during the day as you wish. You do this in any position, lying down, sitting up or standing. It may take a while to really get the hang of it, please be patient.

*Belly to Chest Breath - After you have done the belly breath a number of times, days weeks etc. and it becomes second nature for you, you can begin to invite the breath to rise from the belly up to the chest. Or, you may have noticed this starting to happen naturally. Any of the positions, lying, sitting or standing is fine, but this time hands can be placed both one at the belly and one at the chest. The breath goes into the belly first and then rises upwards until the breast bone (sternum) rises forward from the chest, the chest wall widens out and the collar bones (clavicles) widen moving right and left. Caution, resist the temptation of allowing the shoulders to rise, tighten or move. Encourage them to stay relaxed, remember they are accessory muscles that lift them, not the primary respiratory muscles. Once you fill this space notice if your body is fast to let it go or if you can have a second or two pause before the exhalation. This time releasing the breath from the top of the chest first and the belly last. So, think of filling a glass with liquid, it fills from the bottom to the top. If you are sipping the liquid with a straw the volume would decrease from the top of the glass first and the bottom last. Notice how the breath with naturally elongate the body(especially the trunk) in the inhalation and shorten the body in the exhalation. Try to make the exhalation a few seconds longer than the inhalation, as it is the exhalation that has the most stress and blood pressure reducing benefits.

*Making it 3 Part Breath – After you have done the belly to chest breath a number of times, days weeks etc. and it becomes second nature for you, you can begin to invite the quiet and calm space in. Any of the positions, lying, sitting or standing is fine, and hands can be placed both one at the belly and one at the chest. Continue with the Belly to Chest Breath. Once you fill the lungs from the belly to the chest, find a second or two pause before the exhalation. Notice the sense of calm and peace in that space. Take time to notice any changes and embrace the sensations of quiet. When ready exhale naturally and repeat a number of times. Now, inhale fully but do not pause, exhale and find the pause after the exhalation. Pause for a second or two; give yourself time to notice the quiet and calmness. Continue this for as long as you feel comfortable. When you feel ready begin to find the pause at the end of both the inhalation and exhalation. Noticing the entire breath cycle has now gotten longer and the feeling of release and calm. Use of the 3-part breath is helpful before bed to create a more restful peaceful state. Do notice, if you are holding your breath and feel tension, this breath may not be for you. It is a pause, a brief calm space between, as opposed to a hold that builds tension and pressure.

*Humming – This is another way to find calm but can be uncomfortable when others are around you, as any part of the 3-part breath can be done when alone or around others.

For humming choose the standing or chair sitting position. Following a full deep breath in, with a closed mouth start to hum, this can be a song, or just a humming sound. Notice how the humming begins to lengthen and your mind's direction will turn its focus on the hum moving attention away from what may have been in your thoughts. This also triggers a calming response in the nervous system. The humming produces a vibration in the throat that helps with Vagal tone bringing the body into a more harmonized balance state. Some feel that the hum is the most effective technique for creating calm.

***Deep Breathing** to create focus, strength and an energetic state. The 3-part breath and humming create a sense of calm but there are times where we want to create focus, strength and energy. Like the 3-part breath you can do this lying, sitting, or standing but this breath focuses on the side (lateral) expansion of the rib cage as opposed to the belly. You can use your hands to feel the lower sides of your ribs as they expand out like fish gills with your inhalation and how they come back together when you exhale. In fact, you can connect to the contraction of the abdominal muscles in the exhaling stage and how the fingers of both hands come closer to one another. This breath, although, slow and full has a strong exhale contracting the abdominals and narrowing at the back of the throat creating a sound like the wind. The breath both in and out is done through the nose and you will notice the exhalation to be longer than the inhale, especially now because there is less resistance breathing in, the breath fills easily and fully; where with the exhale we narrow the back of the throat causing a resistance but activating the belly muscles to work supporting and increasing the exhale. There is an added benefit of this breath technique, it helps to loosen up our rib cage which is reliant on mobility but is subject to degenerative arthritic changes decreasing its movement. In order for our lungs to expand fully our rib cage must be able to expand creating space for the lungs.

***Alternate Nostril Breathing** is best done seated. It increases our focus and decision-making capabilities by helping balance the brain's communication. (remember I mentioned nasal laterality?) It doesn't specifically create energy or calm, but when practiced you will forget what was troubling you as you draw focus and attention to doing the breath technique, so a positive byproduct is a more balanced and peaceful state. Ancient yogis considered this breath technique as one to balance the brain. Each hemisphere of the brain has specific qualities: right brain is imagination, intuition, is very creative and emotional and the left brain is more analytical and factual and language skills.

Use your dominant hand to cover both your right and left nostril alternately. (Traditionally it is done using the right hand) First breath is in the left nostril, covering the right nostril for the inhale, then releasing it for the exhale thru the right while covering the left nostril, breathe back into the right nostril keeping the left covered; then exhale thru the left covering the right. That is one cycle in left out right; in right out left, then keep repeating.

Because the hands are busy and you must be completely focused you will find your attention moves away from what was troubling or overwhelming you... Great if you need your mind clear to take in information or under some sort of questioning like a test.

*Deep (Breathing with a Pause, a Hold, and Exhale – to help calm anxiety and help with insomnia. Long slow deep breath to the count of 4, pause the breathing (do not breath in or breath out) to the count of 4, then exhale to count of 8. Repeat. If pausing for 4 is too long and makes you feel uncomfortable, stressed or a sense of breathlessness, shorten the pause to the count of 2 or 3 instead. It is in that pause that we dive into the stillness. And with a long-prolonged exhale we find a sense of release not just emotionally but physically as well. It is in that exhalation we find our heart rate to decrease a bit along with the blood pressure.

Healing is every breath." **Thich Nhat Hanh**

The Mind

How We Are Affected:

An overwhelming sense of fear, from what is going to happen to me, of losing control, fear of losing life's savings, fear of putting a hardship on our family, fear of losing our independence, fear of pain, fear of the effects of the treatment, fear of being in pain, fear of being alone, fear of losing hair and/or our looks and fear of dying. And fear is a calm word, perhaps it really should be terror. Because from the day you get that horrible diagnosis everything is forever changed. This fear will often morph into anxiety and/or depression, insomnia, a feeling of desperation; roaring out of where we may be trying to stuff it, hide it from ourselves and others. We may revisit our life and want to make huge changes, re-evaluate our legacy and future; and sometime there is great anger, and sometimes we may find a greater purpose.

Nothing makes people feel more angry and depressed than being out of control of their life, having to put trust in the hands of others evoking feelings of desperation. We may think of this in terms of happening early in the diagnosis and treatment, but these feelings can surface at any time. Even if a medical remission is achieved, there may be persistent doubt that the remission is real and the fear of relapse overshadowing any sense of joy. Pervading worries that can disrupt sleep and continually keep the body and mind in a fight or flight mode further stressing us mentally and physically. Many people will take anti-anxiety and antidepressant medications, and they can be very helpful, but they do not replace the work that we need to do to find a more hospitable place for our mind and body. When we rely just on the medications we often need to increase dosages or add medicines because our bodies usually become less responsive over time.

The central nervous system has 2 components, the sympathetic (fight or flight) and the parasympathetic (rest and digest). We have the 2 operating all the time to keep our body and organ systems balanced; but when we are in a constant state of stress, and even during our fight during treatment and healing, the sympathetic can go into overdrive. Vagal tone is considered the key to finding the calm and studies are showing how we lose this tone with constant stress. PTSD (post-traumatic stress disorder) is not uncommon with people who sustain a serious injury or illness as the nervous system becomes hypervigilant and hyper responsive. The body responds to stimuli/stress and goes immediately into that stress response and loses the ability to return to calm. This can be triggered by a word, a smell, a sight, a sound or just the body not recognizing that there is no longer an immediate threat. The heart races, we may initially hold our breath, and then begin to shake. We may notice shortness of breath and maybe even chest pain or stomach upset with a sense of doom and discomfort, panic attacks. Insomnia is common with depression and anxiety or it can be a problem of its own.   But persistent insomnia results in sleep deprivation worsening the depression and/or anxiety, the nervous system can no longer regulate it and return to balance. And more studies are coming out how insomnia can cause or worsen heart problems or diabetes. Scarier is that even though medications for sleep will keep you from being awake, they rob you of the normal sleep stages, so we are still not getting the full benefits from the sleep. (I've been dealing with sleep disruption and I so understand why sleep deprivation is used in torture)

Self-esteem and identity really take a hit when we are diagnosed with a life changing or even threatening illness. Perhaps from surgery changing the body, never to return to its previous state, or the deterioration of the body from the disease itself, or the side effects of treatment, or the loss of abilities we once relied on. We need to learn to accept what is and find a way to love ourselves even when we despise what has happened or is happening to ourselves. To still honor ourselves, to care for ourselves lovingly, to forge a new you identify and sometimes having to find new meaning and new purpose in life. This is truly when we let go of the past, what was; be in the present, the now; and look towards the future but without the need to control what will be.

These are not things the docs will tell you about and quite honestly are disconnected to. They can give you the side effects of this and that, offer you medications to handle your complaints or concerns, urge you on by telling you how the therapy is working. But in the end, only you can make the shift. Having the awareness comes first, ceasing to look at ourselves as parts and pieces, and connecting to our wholeness, taking a holistic approach to healing, being our true selves. It is the work we need to do to not just be survivors but "livers"; living, loving, laughing and embrace our beautiful gift of the present. Whether we have many presents ahead or a few. Make each moment count, live it as it is the last for you or maybe for someone else important to you. We only get one shot at that moment.

Being in the technology age we are exposed to more sensory information in one day now than people were in an entire lifetime 50 years ago. This is being bombarded with artificial light 24 hrs. a day, sounds, stimulation and information which has created more stress, anxieties, sleep disorders, physical as well as mental illness and a prevailing sense of not being able to stop thinking, an always active mind. With this sensory overload we are being told how we should feel, think, act, look, and what is going on in the world with all the miseries and hostilities. We can track brain wave activity and we understand the interplay with neurotransmitters and hormones. Mindfulness and meditation can have profound effects on the mental and physical state of anyone. Science has shown how it improves the connections in the brain and lowers the inflammatory factors. But this is not an easy place to find and even harder if trying to find it in crisis. Not everyone will find it quickly; you may want your eyes open and have something to concentrate on or you may want to close your eyes and go deep into silence, or listen to calming sounds that help you relax. Explore and thank yourself for just going there, as just trying something new is stimulating to the brain helping make new brain cells and the myelin sheath that provides smooth transmission on the brain information highway.

So even when you think the big problem is behind you, you get to read this "Patients with diffuse large B cell lymphoma (DLBCL) are at an elevated mortality risk from non-cancer causes even after the disease is cured, according to a study published in Cancer. The greatest increased risk is from blood disease, also increased risk of infection, gastrointestinal disease, vascular diseases, and lung disease. In between 0 and 59 months post-diagnosis were particularly high; after 59 months these risks were lower, though not non-existent." The stress of it all just doesn't disappear, it just takes a back seat the more we are LIVING.

"The Past is History, The Future is a Mystery, The Present is a Gift" Lisa **Unger**

Quieting the Mind - Find Inner Peace and Calm

1. A place to start is just to find quiet and turn off the outside world. Sit quietly listening to calming music or something with natural sounds like the sounds of the ocean, rain, singing birds etc. . . . Sit by water, whether a pond, a lake, the ocean, a water fall or fountain and look into the water, try to breath with each ripple or wave. Sit comfortably with a pet, stroking the pet and notice the breathing. Watch children play. Just come to a place without the technology and just breathe. Be patient as the hardest part is finding quiet within, turning off the endless chatter. Because the mind can only focus on one thing at a time focus on that surrounding.

2. Find a comfortable quiet place, turn off the cell phone, the TV, put pets in another room, try to limit all distractions. Eyes can be open, you can focus on something like a candle flame, or eyes closed visualizing something or with whatever comes up. Maybe what you focused on before that brought you calm put it in your mind's eye. Develop for yourself a mantra, a positive affirmation to repeat to yourself to create new pathways in your brain. If you tend towards anxiety your affirmation could be: "I am feeling calm." "I am feeling strong" You can use an affirmation for healing "I am returning to health" "I am healing". You can say these affirmations out loud, in a whisper or just to yourself. Or do it quietly, in a whisper, out loud, in a whisper and then quietly. Traditional mantras are repeated 108 times as this is thought how many times it takes to form the new neural pathways in the brain. Regardless of whether you do 108 times or not, it must be repeated, so whenever you feel your mind wandering somewhere that isn't beneficial repeat your mantra. (Prayer beads and rosaries are 108 beads used for counting prays) Did you know there are also 108 stitches in a baseball.?

(You may wonder why we don't use an affirmation like "I am not anxious", well, your brain picks up on the I am and leaves out the not. So, in fact, you would be saying to yourself" I am Anxious" reinforcing the very thing you would like to change. So positive affirmations only, not using the negative. Think about the last time you said to yourself "don't forget the keys", and yes, you forgot the keys, so what would have made you remember them would have been "Remember to take the keys".

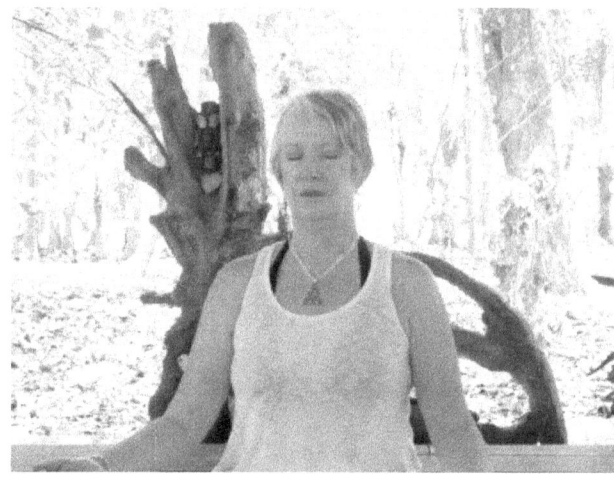

3. One of the most difficult aspects of meditation is not letting the mind wander, fixating on something or being able to just clear the mind to be still. This is called the monkey mind, as our thoughts go from one place to the next like a monkey swinging from tree to tree. Clearing the mind is a skill that needs to be practiced, practiced and practiced; and then not reacting to thoughts that try to intrude, this is mindfulness. The beauty of mindfulness is that it is available to us anywhere, anytime and it can help us in all aspects of our life. A tool for LIVING.

To be mindful is to not attach ourselves to our thoughts, to realize our thoughts are separate from us and to not react to them. Being mindful is to observe the thoughts as being merely thoughts, not reality, and to not react in anyway such as questioning them or try to get in a fight with them like trying to force them out. In fact, the more we react to them, even trying to tell ourselves to stop thinking like that, to try to usher the thoughts out, we are actually strengthening them by putting our attention on them. Our thoughts themselves are benign, it is our reaction to them that gets us into trouble.

"Health is a relationship between you and your body" ~**Terri Guillemets**

"Do not sit still; start moving now. In the beginning, you may not go in the direction you want, but as long as you are moving, you are creating alternatives and possibilities."
Rodolfo Costa, Advice My Parents Gave Me: and Other Lessons I Learned from My Mistakes

The Physical Body

Before I started chemo, I read a study that rats were given chemotherapy and then ran on their wheel. The activity and distribution of the chemo was then measured and they found it increased because of the activity. So, from this I devoted myself to walking especially the days right after chemo and as often as I could to distribute the drugs as much as possible, and with strong breath work to infuse it into every cell. And a gentle therapeutic yoga practice to help settle my mind and find peace with my warrior battle.

If you are fit and active at your diagnosis, staying active throughout your treatment will be much easier. Energy will definitely be impacted, and as time goes on strength may diminish as the muscle mass decreases, flexibility and mobility may be impacted as chemo drugs are very dehydrating to the body causing the connective tissues (ligaments, tendons and cartilage) and fascia to become dry and less pliable. Because chemo drugs affect cell growth, the body will not be able to repair itself if stressed by too much challenge, so all activity needs to be done in moderation, honoring the body's changes and special needs. Body weight exercising like Yoga and Pilates are excellent ways of keeping active and fit. This isn't the time to try to build muscle, endurance or become more conditioned because it's just not going to happen. But stay active, the movement keeps the body more fluid and mobile, helping the healing and restoration of the body and mind. It makes one feel alive, helping with daily activities, and making us more able to withstand the rigors of treatment both physically and mentally. "motion is lotion"

If you do not participate in physical activities prior to treatment, that is not an excuse to not start, in fact your body will respond in positive ways and you will have a head start in living life fully when treatment is done. But do discuss with your medical team your intention for movement activities and get their go ahead before starting. Find someone who is knowledgeable about your medical condition and treatment to guide you and work in conjunction with your medical team. Everything that I present below is to promote more mobility, increase circulation and lymphatic drainage, improve strength, balance and a stronger connection to yourself. "Bodies in motion stay in motion, bodies at rest stay at rest" Einstein's theory of relativity wasn't referring to exercise but nothing could be more appropriate and pertinent.

Let's Start

1. **Breathe** - notice the natural movements of the body in breath, how the trunk (torso) elongates when we breathe in, how the rib cage expands by widening, how the arms move slightly away from the body and how the chin rises slightly. And when we exhale our trunk shortens a bit, our rib cage comes back in, our arms come back down to our sides and the chin drops down a bit. This is the natural/organic movement associated with the breath and this is what yoga is about. Movement emanating from the breath and then allowing a natural expansion with arms, legs, changing of position, etc. In yoga we move slowly and take time to notice. If your breath or body becomes tense or tired, slow down, relax, it isn't a race.

Begin by either sitting in a chair, on a mat with the buttocks raised on a blanket or pillow or standing. From the natural movement begin to expand the elevation of the arms as they move from the body, notice how they rise a bit higher with each breath and then return to the body on the exhale. As the arms and shoulders begin to free, the arms can begin to reach upward at the crest of the inhalation and then return slowly to the body at the end of the exhale. Noticing how the trunk continues to lengthen and the chest widens when the arms are extended out. Feel the chest expand more and more with each inhale, as the breath deepens and lengthens.

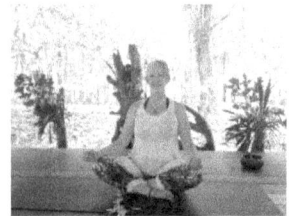 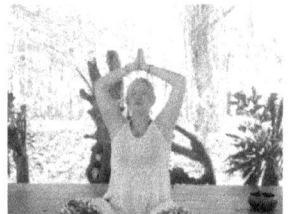 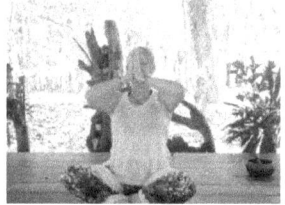 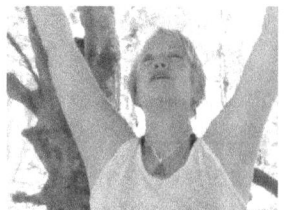

Once the arms can comfortably reach to the sky, turning the palms to face one another raised just above the shoulders, feel the shoulders relax down with the exhale. Hold this for a few breaths, notice how the sides of the body lengthen and we open up all the neglected spaces in our bodies. Do not hold your breath, keep the breath long, slow and deep. If the breath gets short and tight, relax the arms, noticing our breath is the best way to see if we are working too hard or just right.

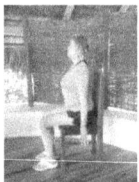 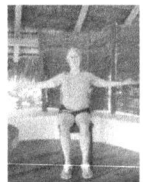 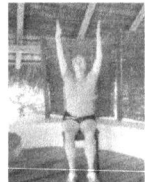 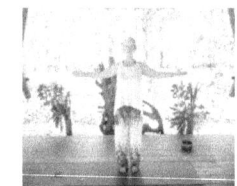 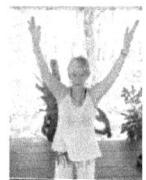

> *"Take care of your body. It's the only place you have to live."* **Jim Rohn**

2. Movement - as we noticed how the body moves naturally with the breath we begin to create purposeful movement from the breath. *(When we are frightened, angry, depressed, anxious or in pain we tighten our neck and drop our chin down, letting our shoulders roll forward, and eventually the back becomes tight and movement becomes more difficult. Our goal to movement is to help keep us open and moving freely)* One of the most beneficial movements is for spinal, specifically thoracic mobility. Not only will it help relieve back and shoulder tension, pain, tightness and stress, but it will help open the lungs by creating more space and toning the respiratory muscles, improving respiration, decreasing fatigue and shortness of breath.

*From a seated position (preferably a hardback chair without arms), with arms softly to our sides, as we inhale turn our hands open with palms up and thumbs pointing back and start to extend arms out and open without raising them very much. Feel the chest wall/the breast bone lift upwards and forward, as we begin to exhale let the hands come back towards the front of the body with hands gently touching, overlapping like a hug or just coming near one another by the lap. Repeat as the movements grow, the breath deepens and the body loosens. Notice how the body begins to open up, our arms may begin to rise a little higher and we begin to release any tension of mind or body. The natural movements begin to flow, openness with the air moving in and release as the air moves out. Effortless, organic, calming but yet enlivening. Paying attention not to lift the arms with the top of the shoulders, keeping the shoulders and neck relaxed and letting the arms feel as though they are floating.

As this movement begins to feel more natural, comfortable and we can feel the freeing of our body and mind, linger in the open position for a few breaths. Let the hands reach back to connect to the chair back. Not holding the breath but diving beneath the surface to find the still space beneath. Making sure the shoulders are relaxed, our chest is expanded, nothing is forced and we can feel our body making space for the breath. Remembering the movement follows the breath, it is natural/organic, fostering growth and positive change.

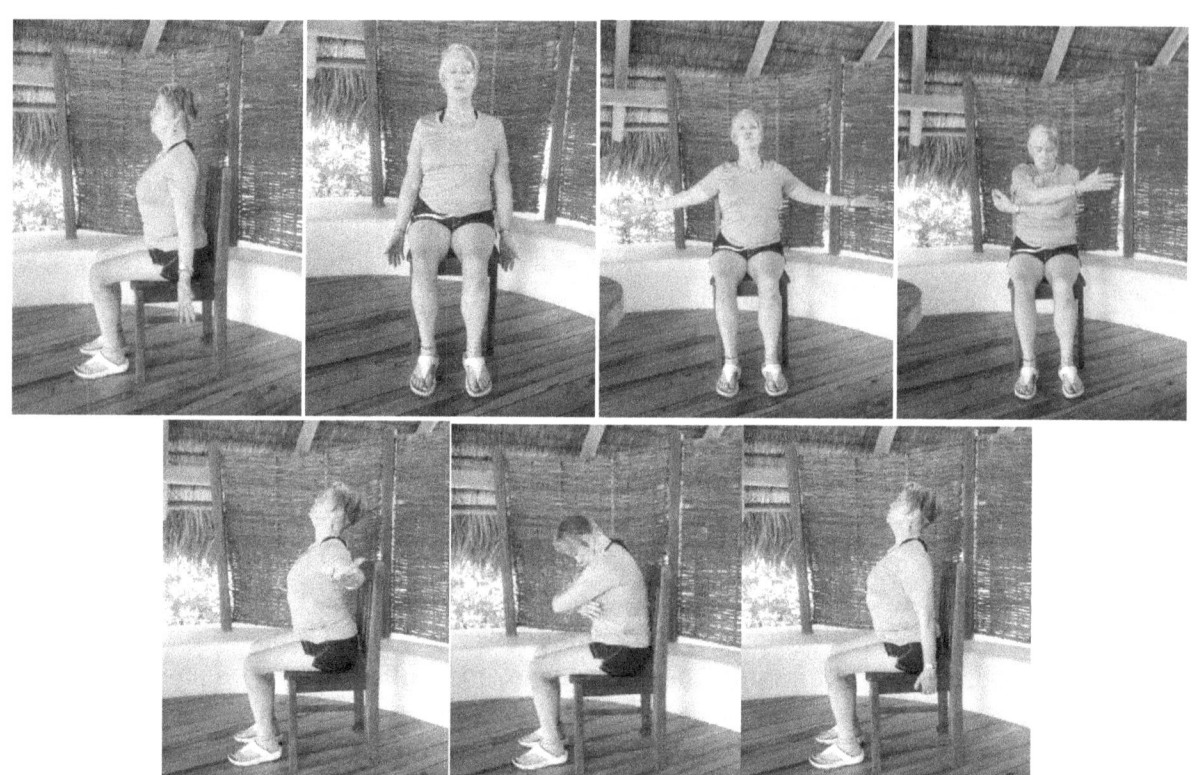

*When you feel ready to go further, but never rush, there is no race: The next step is to come to the forearms and knees. Elevating the forearms with a folded blanket or towel until you are not feeling a downward force at the upper body   Find a comfortable hand position, as the hands can come together and just the outer edge (ulna aspect) of the hands are on the mat, let the hands have a comfortable space between them or let the forearms and palms come down on the ground. Making sure there is no pinching or tightness in the shoulders, as the forearms press into the ground making us feel lifted as opposed to our body feeling heavy on the forearms. Making sure there is sufficient padding under the knees and forearms. Alignment and support are important as the hips align over the knees but let the knees separate to a comfortable position, the toes can be pointed or curled under, whichever feels the most supportive, and without discomfort; the shoulders align over the elbows. The energy of the body is lifted with the breath so that the body doesn't weigh heavy on the forearms, in fact the forearms energetically press into the ground giving the body lift.   With the inhalation the tail bone points skyward and the chest cascades upward with the head lifting being careful not to throw the head back. The back softens into the chest as the chest lengthens and expands, feeling the shoulder blades slide down the back in towards the spine. As the body is ready to exhale firm the belly muscles without squeezing the buttocks and feel the tail bone begin to point downwards towards the mat. And the movement cascades up the spine, the back lengthens and widens, the shoulder blades move away from the spine into the sides and the forehead points down to the ground.

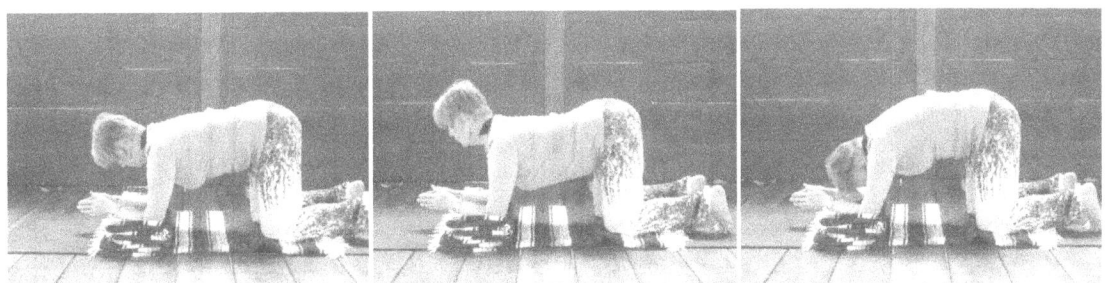

*To increase and advance the movement come to hands and knees. Making sure there is sufficient padding under the knees and hands. Alignment and support are important as the hips align over the knees allowing the knees to be a comfortable distance apart, the toes can be pointed or curled under, whichever feels the most supportive, and without discomfort; the shoulders align over the wrists, make sure the fingers are spread wide and the arches of the hands are not pressed down. Feel the rim of the hands contacting the ground, stretch and widen the fingers with your focus towards the web space between the thumb and index finger. The energy of the body is lifted with the breath so that the body doesn't weigh heavy on the wrists. With the inhalation the tail bone points skyward and the chest cascades upward with the head lifting avoiding tilting the head backwards. The back softens into the chest as the chest lengthens and expands, feeling the shoulder blades slide down the back in towards the spine. As the body is ready to exhale firm the belly muscles without squeezing the buttocks and feel the tail bone begin to point downwards towards the mat. And the movement cascades up the spine the back lengthens and widens, the shoulder blades move away from the spine into the sides and the forehead points down to the ground. The movement can flow letting each breath create more space and fluidity in the body. As the movement becomes easier and any tightness begins to loosen, stay in each of the positions for a few breaths, keeping the shoulders away from the ears and not pushing or straining. Let the natural breath create the expansion and relaxation.

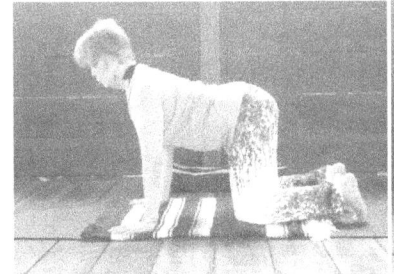 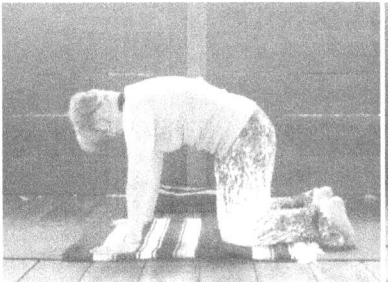 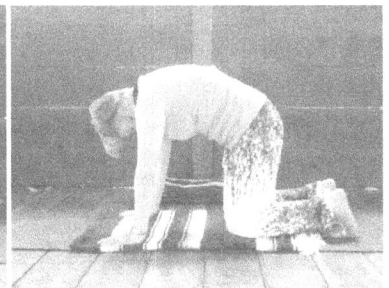

*As the body begins to loosen and the movement flows with the breath gently turn your head to one side with the inhale and exhaling back into the rounding/lengthening/widening of the back with the head back to neutral, then repeat to the other side with the inhale, feeling the shift in weight and focus. Drawing awareness to the connection to the abdominal wall as the weight shifts. Noticing that without tension in the shoulders and the neck the head turns with ease. Keeping the head in line with the spine looking forward and out in the inhale and looking down with the exhale recentering.

*As this movement becomes easier and the body continues to create more space bring your hip to the side you are looking creating a little side bend. Repeat this in a flowing fashion allowing the exhale to deepen the side bending move and using the inhale to return to the center then repeat to the opposite side. Flow in and out of this a few times and then settle yourself into the bend, pausing the body but feeling the expansion of the longer side with the breath. Linger there for a few breaths feeling the opening of the rib cage, the lengthening of the space between the hip and shoulder, maybe even letting the hips ease back towards the heels a bit to work into it a little more. When ready come back to center and repeat to the opposite side.

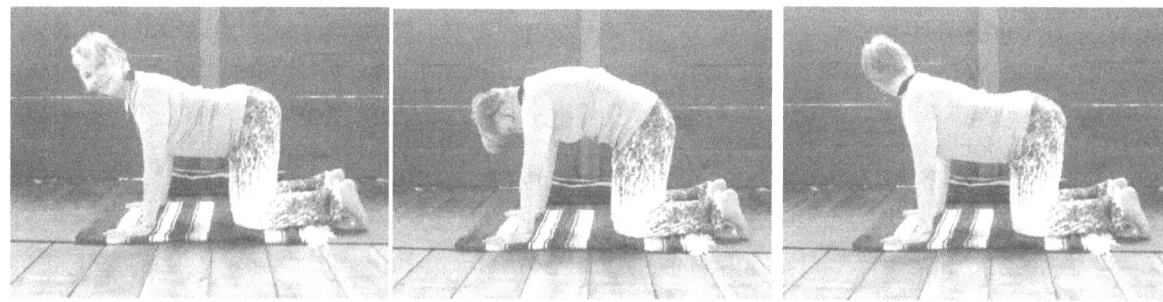

Take time to notice not just the loosening, lengthening, stretching and freeing of the body but notice the sense of calming. Taking the time to nurture ourselves, to listen, create an inner massage all the while improving our breath, our muscles, bones, and joints, finding that inner strength and connection. Letting our bodies follow our inner compass, our breath taking us on a journey to a happier and calmer state of well-being.

As we begin to add standing movement to help with strength and balance, take care to provide a safe space, having a chair available for support and to sit on if there is any dizziness or sense of weakness. When we can stand strong on our own 2 feet we re-establish ourselves, connect and be one in breath, mind and body.

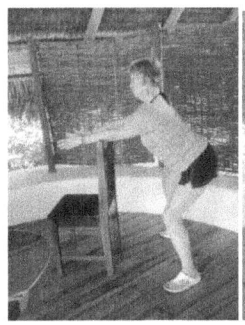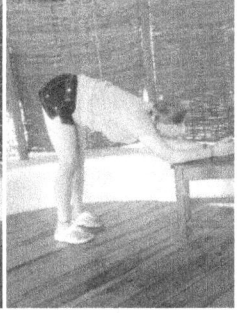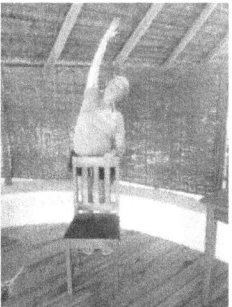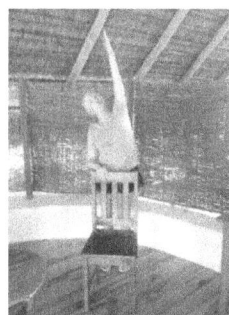

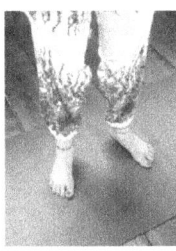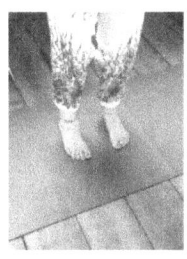

> You may notice that all the standing poses are done barefoot. It is not required but because the feet give us our grounding and balance there is more information transmitted and received by the nervous system barefoot. Shoes do alter how your foot meets the earth. But do what is most comfortable and safe for you.

*Take a moment to find a standing position, let the legs widen a bit to align under the hips to create more balance. At first the toes may turn out so that the body can have more stability. As your standing becomes stronger try to start bringing the feet a little closer in with less turn out of the toes. With neuropathy of the feet your stance will automatically be a little wider to accommodate for the lack of sensation and feedback from the feet on the ground. At first the chair back can be directly in front so that one or both hands can hold it for support. As the sense of balance and strength increases move the arms softly to our sides. Adjust the shoulders so that the palms are turning to the front (thumbs pointing away from the body). Shift the weight forward more onto the balls of the feet and then back onto the heels lifting the toes upward, and shift to the sides of the feet noticing changes in the legs, our core/trunk and head. Notice if you are standing heavier on one side or the other. Find a strong standing position with the knees playfully released (not pushing into the knee joints) and feel the muscles of the legs firm into the bones, the head is held high, shoulders relaxed and we just breathe into our body connecting to its sensations, natural rhythm and movements.

*As you begin to feel strong in our stance, not needing to hold on, as we inhale turn our hands open with palms up and thumbs pointing back and start to extend arms out and open, without lifting the arms. Feel the chest wall/the breast bone lift upwards and forward, as we begin to exhale let the hands come back towards the front of the body with hands gently touching, overlapping like a hug or just coming near one another allowing the arms to raise where it feels natural. Effortless, organic, calming but yet enlivening. Paying attention not to lift the arms with the top of the shoulders, keeping the shoulders and neck relaxed and letting the arms feel as though they are floating.

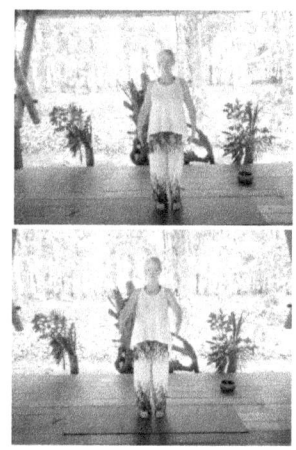 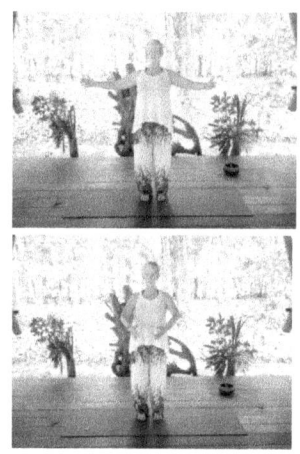 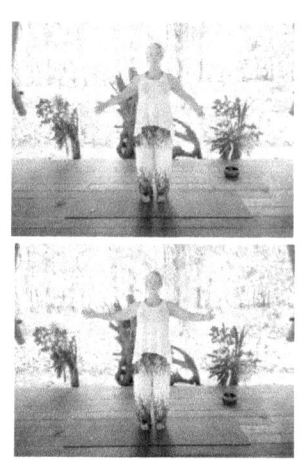

Allow this movement to become natural, free and comfortable, linger in the open position for a few breaths. Not holding the breath but feeling the quiet, diving beneath the surface to find the still space of calmness. Making sure the shoulders are relaxed, nothing is forced and we can feel our body making space with the breath. Remembering the movement follows the breath, it is natural/organic fostering growth and positive change. In this standing flowing movement, as our body may begin to free and move with a flowing action we may feel our entire body letting go of stress, worry, tension and even pain.

*Since our shoulders respond to our stress by getting tight and traveling upwards towards our ears, making us feel as though we are truly carrying the weight of the world on us, it is important to allow freedom of movement, the sensation of letting go of that tension before raising the arms up over the head. If we are holding lots of tension in our shoulder and neck and have been using just the upper half of our lungs, overhead movements can cause more tension. Once we are noticing the difference in our breathing and in the movement of our rib cage, we can begin to focus on raising the arms to create more length as well as more lung space. As you begin, you may want to face a mirror to see if your shoulders come up to the ears, as tension has us lift that way. Or you can ask someone to assist you, placing their hands on the top of your shoulders giving you feed back as you begin the movement.

*Beginning in a strong standing position, you can use a chair back to hold with one hand for support or keep one hand down touching your outer thigh or hip, raise the other hand as you inhale by turning the palm upwards, raising the arm from the side until the arm is straight up, fingers reaching to the sky. As you begin to exhale let the arm retrace the same plane of motion with the palm returning to rest at the hip or outer thigh. Repeat that same side a few times, then do the other side. As you feel the connection to the movement, the arm rising up with the inhale and the arm floating back down with the exhale, begin a small reach over as you increase the length in the side of the body with the extended arm. As you repeat this alternating sides, stay in the pose, relaxing the shoulders and breathing into the space and length of the raised side. Feel *the body going a little further into the move as the breath dictates. Notice the balance at the feet and legs, trying to keep the hips firm and strong not sway.*

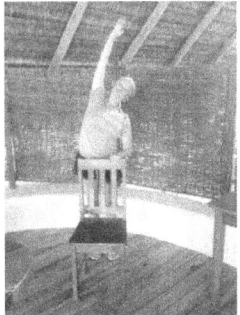
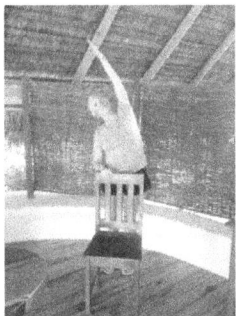

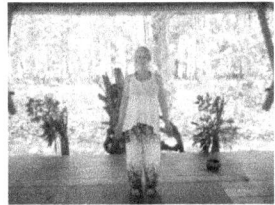
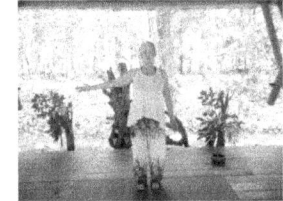
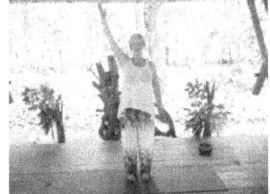

*As you are ready to increase the movement and body challenge begin moving both arms out and up with the inhale until the fingers are pointing to the sky. Keep one arm up, lower the opposite arm with the exhale coming into a small side bend to the side of the arm coming down. With the next inhalation coming out of the side bend and raising the arm back up until both arms are raised stretching reaching and lengthening. Repeat to the opposite side, holding the side bend as it feels comfortable, feet and legs strong without swaying the hips to either side.

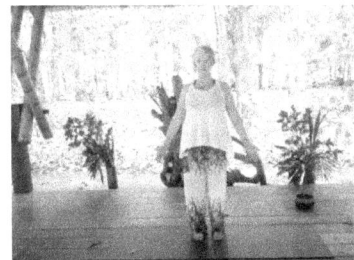
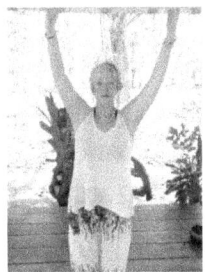
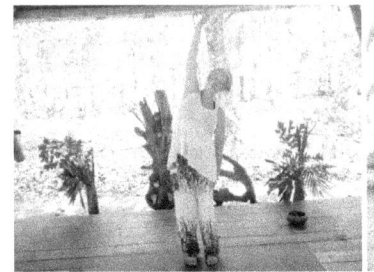
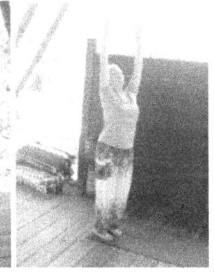

As we move our upper body we start to notice our center of gravity, where we feel grounded and strong and when our movement becomes larger and challenges that stable base. Even with 2 feet on the ground we can notice our balance being challenged. The standing side bends can be modified being done while sitting in a chair. Make sure both feet are firmly on the ground as you sit in a hard-back chair, allow the hand that is down to slide down the chair leg. Do not let the hand dangle, give the hand purpose and let it make a connection which will confer strength and safety with the movement and balance. Even sitting on the chair, you will notice the center of gravity at the pelvis, try to keep both butt cheeks on the chair with the side bend creating space in the side body and finding balance as opposed to just moving your body weight to one side.

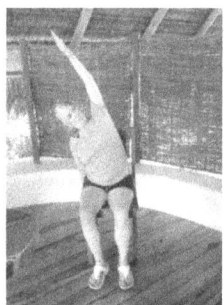 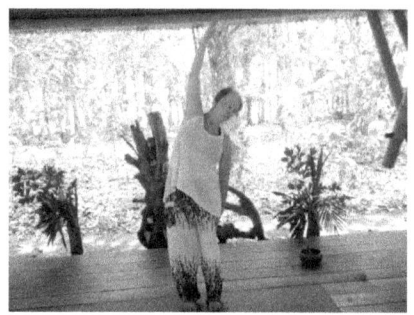

Movement, whether we are speaking about the entire body, spine or extremities is multi-directional. So, movements that just concentrate on forward and back and/or side to side movements are not sufficient. We must incorporate twisting. Twists help to squeeze out tension of the muscles, the joints, see things from a different perspective, and allowing the body to move in other directions more fully and freely. Twists, though, can be thought of as a progression, so that is why I am incorporating them at the end of my suggested movements. Done standing or seated the benefits can be noticed in increased movement and flexibility immediately after.

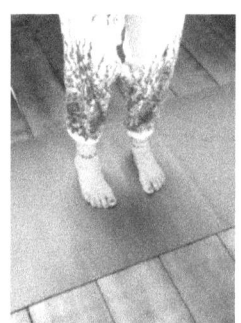 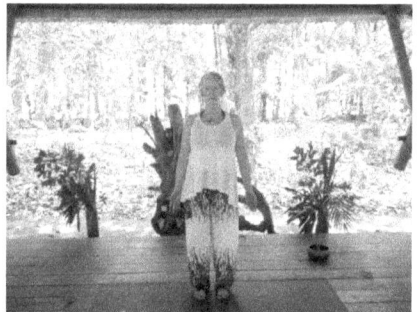

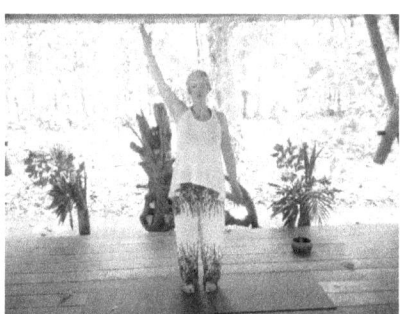 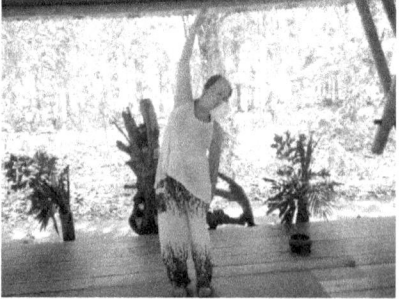

Twists can be done seated or standing. For standing begin with your feet in a strong grounded position, feet hip width apart and toes pointing forward. The twisting movement should be done with the body in a lengthened position, so do a few raises of the arms first to feel the spine lengthen with the head reaching up to the sky. Once in that long-lengthened position turn the upper body only, the hips stay facing forward and weight shared equally on both feet. Shoulders stay relaxed, hand opposite to the direction of the twist (contra lateral side) crosses the front of the body going to the hip on the twist side, and the hand on the same side of the twist (ipsilateral side) comes down to the leg and slightly posterior. As long as the shoulders stay in a depressed/relaxed position, the turning side hand (ipsilateral side) can move behind the back toward the opposite hip. If you begin to feel any tension, tightness, discomfort or strain in that shoulder, arm or neck lower the hand back down to its same side thigh. To take it a bit deeper the arm that is crossed in front at the hip came move up to that shoulder as long as the shoulder doesn't hike upwards. Breathe into the body, elongating the spine, expanding the chest, relaxing the shoulders and deepen into the twist a bit more as your body invites. Caution about the neck, allow the head to remain in a neutral alignment, facing the direction of the breast bone. If you want a little twist in the neck, allow the head to gaze in the direction of the twist after the body has settled into it for a few breaths. Turning the head too much can cause dizziness and strain so pay attention to what you are experiencing/feeling, this isn't a race. Come out of the twist slowly and pause for a few breaths before twisting to the opposite side. Now see how both sides feel, notice if there is any tightness, restriction, which side has more twisting, if your breath feels less full on one side as opposed to the other. In this case either spend a little more time in the more challenged side or repeat that side one additional time allowing you to work more there.

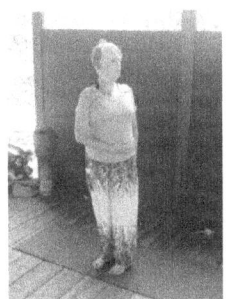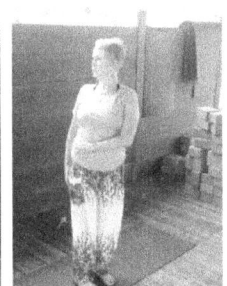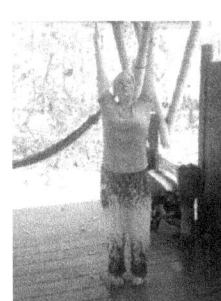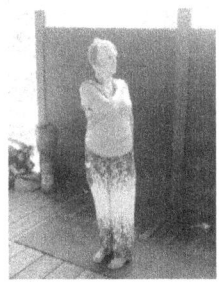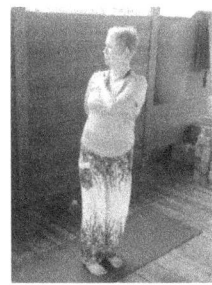

Seated twists, done while sitting in a chair with both feet firmly on the ground as you sit in a hard-back chair. Even sitting on the chair, you will notice the center of gravity at the pelvis, elongating the spine and try to keep both butt cheeks on the chair with the twist creating space in the body and finding balance. The hand opposite to the direction of the twist (contra lateral side) goes to the thigh on the side of the twist. The hand on the side of the twist slides down the chair leg (instead of your thigh in standing). Do not let the hand dangle, give the hand purpose and let it make a connection which will confer strength with the movement and balance. When you want to deepen the twist, you can bring your arm over the back of the chair letting the hand rest into the back of the chair and the opposite hand moves closer towards the hip. Come out of the twist slowly and pause for a few breaths before twisting to the opposite side. Now see how both sides feel, notice if there is any tightness, restriction, which side has more twisting, if your breath feels less full on one side as opposed to the other. In this case either spend a little more time in the more challenged side or repeat that side one additional time allowing you to work more there.

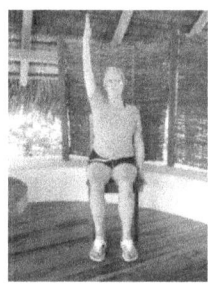 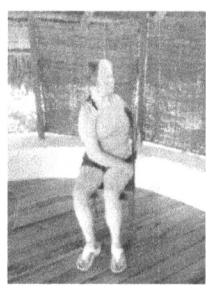 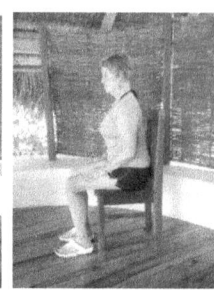 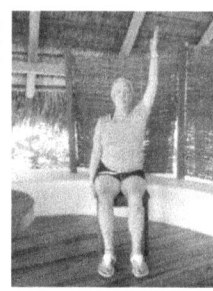 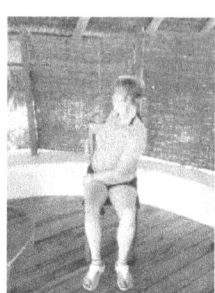

As you progress, I recommend doing the side bends before the twisting and then repeating the side bends again. The difference is immediately noticeable and you will become more attuned to your body, knowing what it is you need and how far you can go safely and effectively.

And then take some time to return to just breath, to be quiet, notice what there is to notice. Don't be afraid to breath, to move, to feel. Fear paralyzes us, will restrict us and numb us. Explore and do these as often as you want, and watch transformations taking place. There is so much more but we have to start somewhere. Please check out my Facebook for tips, tools and inspiration.

This book is not a substitute for medical care and guidance. And share with your medical providers any information and tools for their approval before undertaking them.

This Isn't the End

And so, I close this writing, I am hoping the story and helpful ideas can go on and on and on for a long time, but I need to have a jumping off point for the book. I am traveling as much as I can, telling people that instead of planning vacation around work, I now plan work around vacation. I want to celebrate everyday as if it is a holiday, because for me it is a day for celebration. Every morning I wake up with gratitude, I express gratitude for my health, my wellness, my happiness, my wholeness, my life, and the love that is given to me and I can give to others.

My present is life and what an amazing gift it is. Thank you, thank you, thank you for taking the time to read this book. I hope you have found it insightful, inspiring and helpful. Has given you some smiles, laughter and tears. Life is a roller coaster, be on it for the fun of it.

Thank you to my wonderful husband, John, who is so proud to see me soar after such a big life challenge for myself, for him and for our relationship. And a thank you to my amazing son Nick who never doubted in the success of my LIVING. Both of them participating in taking my photos with my phone's camera.

A big wow to Boca Sombrero Yoga & Beach Resort in Puerto Jimenez, Costa Rica for providing such a beautiful, peaceful, natural getaway and to Ginger Garner having the Professional Yoga Therapy Institute Retreat for me to participate in and for the inspiring photo and creative opportunity. I began this venture at the retreat in 2016 so it was where I wanted to bring the pictorial essence together in 2017. And a big yay to Royal Caribbean Cruises where I spent lots of my time crossing the Atlantic in my cabin in 2016, 2017 and 2018 writing, editing, proofing, putting this creation together. I am not a writer, wow this is hard work. Respect so much respect to writers.

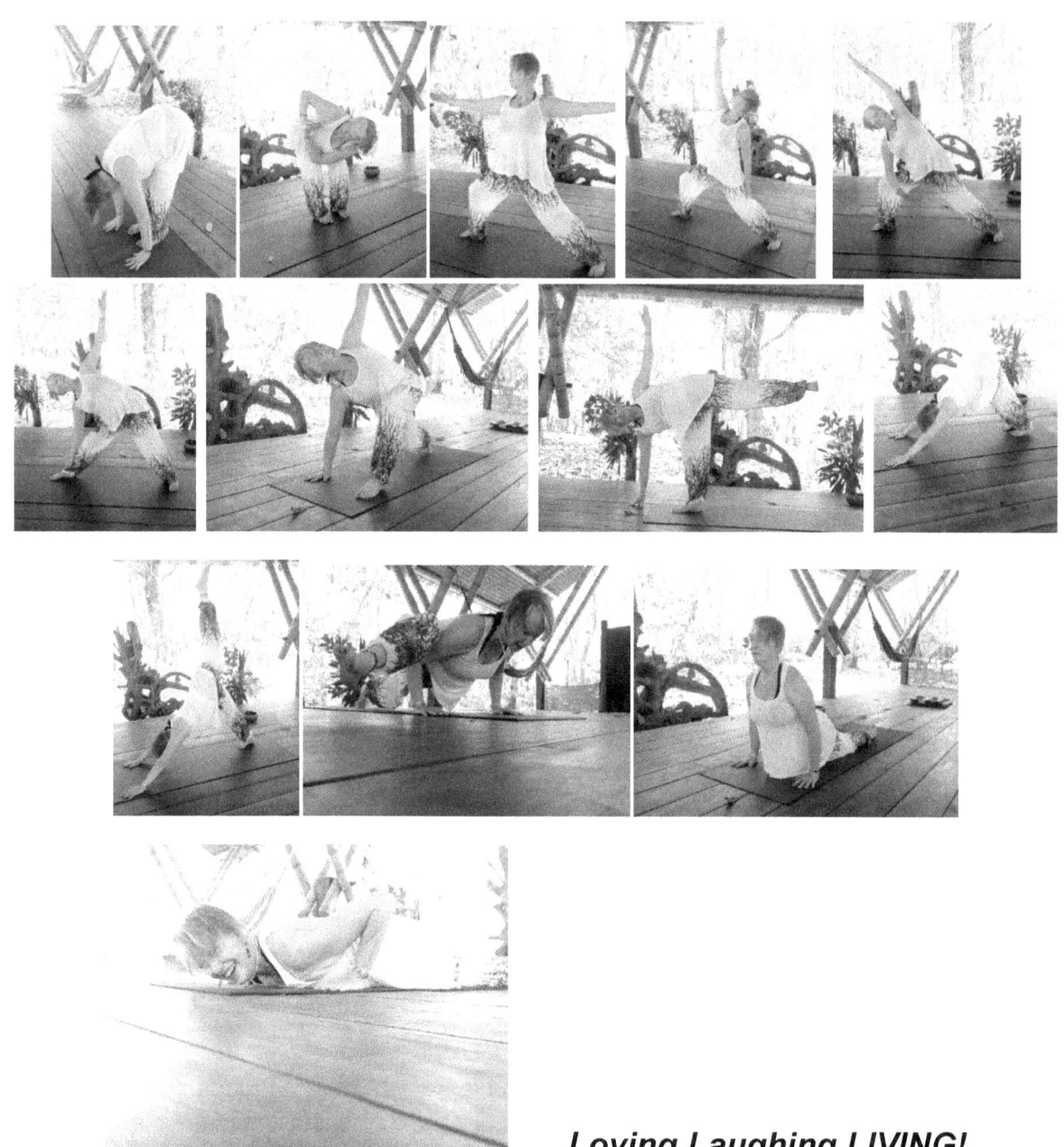

Loving Laughing LIVING!

"Yesterday is history. Tomorrow is a mystery. Today is a gift. That's why it's called the present."
Alice Morse Earle

A portion of the proceeds for this book will be donated to The Leukemia & Lymphoma Society, as they have been an unending source of information, research and support.   www.lls.org

Follow Me On:

Facebook   https://www.facebook.com/Flow-Yoga-Faith-885322668332839

Instagram   https://www.instagram.com/flowyogafaith/

http://www.flowyoga.biz

This book is not a substitute for medical care, guidance and scrutiny. And share with your medical providers any information and tools for their approval before undertaking them.